THE

AAMT

BOOK OF STYLE

FOR MEDICAL TRANSCRIPTION

Claudia Tessier, CAE, CMT, RRA
Executive Director, AAMT

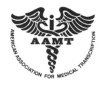

American Association for Medical Transcription
Modesto, California

American Association for Medical Transcription
A Nonprofit Professional Corporation
PO Box 576187, Modesto, California 95357-6187
3460 Oakdale Road, Suite M, Modesto, CA 95355-9691
Phone: 209-551-0883 or 800-982-2182
Fax: 209-551-9317

The AAMT Book of Style for Medical Transcription

ISBN 0-935229-22-1

Printed in the United States of America.

Last digit indicates print number: 10 9 8 7 6 5 4 3 2

Design and layout by Lori Smith.

Printing and binding by Baker Graphics, Riverbank, California.

Dedication

To all medical transcriptionists, most especially to those who place quality before quantity and who practice medical transcription as both an art and a science. This one's for you.

Contents

Introduction vii

A Note to Users of This Book ix

Acknowledgments xi

A–Z entries 1

Appendices 383

About the Author 517

About AAMT 519

Introduction

As the professional association for medical transcription, AAMT is the recognized leader in acknowledging and establishing medical transcription styles, forms, and practices. We communicate these to our members, to other medical transcriptionists, to supervisors and managers, to educators and students, and to the wider healthcare community through our periodicals, publications, modules, videos, and conferences, as well as through direct contact via correspondence, telephone conversations, and in-person meetings, both formal and informal.

This book presents and represents AAMT's most complete conclusions for a wide variety of medical transcription styles, forms, and practices. We acknowledge that there are forms, styles, and practices which differ from those that we have identified, established, and promulgated. We address some alternative forms to demonstrate why we do not prefer them. When we consider two or more alternative forms to be equally acceptable, we indicate this. Where there are no alternatives (in the expression of the symbol *pH,* for example), we state this in the text. Otherwise, we address few alternative forms because, with increased confidence in our knowledge and judgment and with our expanded acceptance as the leader in making these judgments, we prefer to emphasize our conclusions rather than to refute those of others.

We reach our conclusions through research and experience and logic and common sense and through the experience and expertise of MTs within and beyond our membership. We consult other sources, such as the AMA and Associated Press style manuals, but because such references speak to different applications (manuscripts and newspapers, for example), we weigh and consider their conclusions in light of the realities of dictation and transcription, and we adopt, adapt, or reject them accordingly. Likewise, when we consult other MT references, we weigh and consider their conclusions in light of both their and our experience and expertise. Frequently, we resolve inconsistencies among and within such references.

Style is not an exact science. Like dictionaries, style manuals change over time, not only by adding new material but also by revising old material, based on expanding knowledge and experience as well as changing usage and meaning. AAMT's conclusions are themselves scrutinized (by us and others), and when we deem it appropriate we make revisions. For example, in AAMT's previous style reference (*Style Guide for Medical Transcription*), we presented our conclusion that sentences should not begin with an abbreviation. After reconsidering this matter, we now acknowledge that sentences may (and sometimes should) begin with an abbreviation (but not one beginning with a lowercased letter). We changed our conclusion because we recognized that requiring a sentence to be recast to avoid its beginning with an abbreviation may interfere with, rather than enhance, communication and that such construction is so common that it is as readily accepted by the reader as by the listener.

You may wonder what place your personal stylistic decisions and usage should have in your practice of medical transcription. We urge you and other MT practitioners, students, teachers, supervisors, dictators, and others to adopt our forms, styles, and practices, but we take the role of persuader not enforcer. AAMT's conclusions are widely accepted because our reputation for quality and exactness has established us as the recognized leader in the world of medical transcription. By incorporating our conclusions into your practices, you have our expertise and reputation on which to justify your decisions and our materials with which to document them. Those who choose to use styles, forms, and practices other than those promoted by AAMT have a professional obligation to assure that their choices are appropriate, acceptable, and consistent and to be prepared to provide rationale and documentation to substantiate their choices.

A Note to Users of This Book

No style book is ever finished or complete. Something more could be said about each of the topics covered. What has been said could perhaps be said better if said differently. Additional topics could be covered. Perhaps some topics could be deleted. The content could be reorganized. Additional editorial tweaking could improve the presentation.

The temptations and reasons for extending manuscript preparation time are endless. Nevertheless, there comes a time when the decision must be made that a book is ready for publication—or it will be in preparation forever. That time has come for the first edition of *The AAMT Book of Style for Medical Transcription.*

> ## *We are all apprentices in a craft where no one ever becomes a master.*
> Ernest Hemingway

This new style book was only a gleam in AAMT's eye when we published our first style book, *Style Guide for Medical Transcription,* in 1985. Even then, we knew that there was more, much more, to be said about medical transcription styles, forms, and practices. *The AAMT Book of Style for Medical Transcription* demonstrates how right we were. With more than five times the number of pages than the old style guide, it covers many more topics—so many more that we organized it in A-to-Z fashion, with numerous cross-references and appendices, to facilitate the user's quick and easy access to the topics of immediate interest. Or it can be read cover to cover. Or it can be opened at random. Equally at home in the classroom and the workplace, it can serve as a textbook as well as a reference book. All in all, *The AAMT Book of Style for Medical Transcription* will carry AAMT's gold standard for medical transcription further and with greater impact than any previous AAMT publication.

With an audience that includes more than a few who will go to the wall over a comma, we expect that *The AAMT Book of Style for Medical*

Transcription will stimulate not only interest and delight but also controversy. No one will agree with everything in it; too many alternative acceptable forms exist. Many will disagree with one thing or another in it. Such is the nature of style in general and medical transcription in particular—for that matter, such is the nature of people in general and medical transcriptionists in particular.

We ask that you pass on to us your suggestions, questions, comments, and criticisms so that we can consider your input as we prepare the book's second edition. Just as your input was vital to preparing this first edition, we need your input for the next round.

Yes, the second edition of *The AAMT Book of Style for Medical Transcription* is already a gleam in AAMT's eye. It will update topics in this first edition, it will cover an even wider range of topics, and it will address new topics that we can't even predict at this time. Your input will be essential in determining just where and what changes and additions should be made.

So, keep those cards and letters coming, folks. We look forward to your part in ensuring that *The AAMT Book of Style for Medical Transcription* will get better and better, and bigger and bigger, with each edition.

Send inquiries and comments to:

AAMT Book of Style
PO Box 576187
Modesto, CA 95357-6187
Fax: 209-551-9317

Acknowledgments

The whole is truly greater than the sum of its parts. This book wouldn't be—couldn't be—all that it is without the efforts of all those who helped along the way. I share with all those identified below the responsibility for all that is right about this book; as its author, I accept responsibility for any errors, inconsistencies, and shortcomings that it may yet exhibit.

Thanks to the AAMT board and the AAMT staff for their encouragement and support and assistance, as well as for sharing the load that I would, from time to time, set aside in order to work on the manuscript.

Thanks especially to the CMTs on AAMT's staff—Linda Byrne, CMT; Pat Forbis, CMT; Diane Heath, CMT; and Terri Wakefield, CMT—who shared their experience and expertise and editorial eyes and valuable time to review and critique the manuscript, again and again. Without their commitment and caring, this book and AAMT would be greatly diminished.

Very special thanks to Lori Smith, AAMT's director of publications, for her work in the design and layout of the book. She is truly our artist-in-residence.

Thanks to reviewers Martha Ladner, CMT; Carrie Boatman, CMT; Marilyn Craddock, CMT, RRA; and to proofreader David Mitchnick, for their time and expertise. Each brought a different perspective to the process, and because they did, the book is better than it could have been without them.

Thanks to my family and friends, most especially my husband, David Bryon, for encouraging and supporting me in this task even though it meant taking numerous weekends and evenings away from them to do so.

Finally, and most importantly, thanks to all AAMT members and other medical transcriptionists who contributed to this book through their expertise and inquiries. To them and to all who will use this book, I say, **Do it with style!**

Claudia Tessier, CAE, CMT, RRA
Modesto, California
August 1994

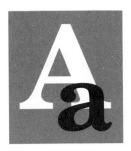

a, an
Indefinite articles. Compare *the*.

before consonants, h's, u sounds, vowels
Use *a* before a consonant, a sounded (aspirate) *h,* or a long *u* sound.
Use *an* before a vowel or an unsounded *h.* The pronunciation of an
abbreviation or a numeral determines whether it is preceded by *a* or *an*.

    a patient
    a hemorrhoid
    a unit
    an indication
    an hour
    a 1-mile run
    an 8-hour delay
    a CMT
    an MD

    See articles

AAMT
Abbreviation for American Association for Medical Transcription.
Usually pronounced as a word (*ampt*) but may be pronounced as a series
of single letters (*A-A-M-T*).

    See American Association for Medical Transcription

AB, BA
Abbreviations for *Bachelor of Arts* degree.

See
bachelor's degree
degrees, academic

abbreviations

Abbreviations in medical dictation are intended to speed up communication, but they frequently create confusion instead. While the dictator may think that dictating the abbreviation *AML* is the fastest way to communicate *acute myelocytic leukemia,* medical transcriptionists know better. They face the dilemma: Does *AML* mean acute monocytic leukemia, acute myeloblastic leukemia, acute myelocytic leukemia, acute myelogenous leukemia, acute myeloid leukemia, or perhaps even some less common alternative? In the numerous publications devoted to translating medical abbreviations, those with a single meaning appear to be in the minority.

For years there was a widespread misunderstanding that JCAHO (the Joint Commission on Accreditation of Healthcare Organizations) had established an official list of abbreviations and that only abbreviations on this list could be used in healthcare records. Let us clarify this misunderstanding. There is no list established or approved by JCAHO, and JCAHO has no requirement or standard related to abbreviations. (Historical note: JCAHO standards used to state that each hospital must prepare its own list of acceptable abbreviations, that only abbreviations on that list should appear in that institution's healthcare records, and that only one meaning should be allowed per abbreviation. JCAHO no longer stipulates even that requirement.)

abbreviating terms dictated in full

Do not abbreviate terminology dictated in full except for units of measurement, e.g., "milligrams," "centimeters," etc. Such abbreviations are universally known and accepted and may even be used in diagnostic statements or operative titles, for they are not themselves the diagnosis or operation name. Indeed, abbreviated forms are preferable because they communicate their meaning more quickly and succinctly than their extended forms.

abbreviations with multiple meanings

What should an MT do when an abbreviated diagnosis, conclusion, or operative title is dictated and the abbreviation has multiple meanings? In the best of scenarios, either the physician will use the extended term else-where in the dictation or the content of the report will somehow make the extended term obvious. Further, the MT will have equipment that allows insertion of the full term wherever the abbreviation is dictated, without the need to re-keyboard the entire document.

When confronted with less than the best of scenarios, if there is easy and immediate access to the patient's record or the dictating physician, the MT can determine the meaning from one or the other. Without such access, the best the MT can do is use the abbreviation (or leave a blank) and attach a note asking the dictator to enter the intended meaning on the report. If even the abbreviation is not understandable (ANL? AML? ANO? AMO?), the MT has no choice but to leave a blank and flag the report.

> ### *There is a profound difference between information and meaning.*
> Warren G. Bennis

at beginning of sentence

It is increasingly acceptable, often preferable, to begin a sentence with a dictated abbreviation, acronym, or brief form (except units of measure). Of course, it is also acceptable to write it out.

WBC was 9200.
or White blood count was 9200.

Exam was delayed.
or Examination was delayed.

in diagnoses and operative titles

Write out the abbreviation in full if the abbreviation is used in the admission, discharge, preoperative, or postoperative diagnosis; consul-tative conclusion; or operative title. These are critical points of informa-tion, and their meanings must be clear to assure accurate communication for patient care, reimbursement, statistical, and medicolegal documen-tation. Elsewhere in reports, i.e., within the narrative portions, common and readily understood abbreviations may be transcribed if dictated, or they may be written in full. Other abbreviations should be transcribed in full.

If unable to translate the abbreviation, the MT should transcribe it as dictated or leave a blank and then flag the report, asking the dictator to translate it.

Non-disease entity abbreviations accompanying diagnostic and procedure statements may be used if dictated, e.g., abbreviated units of measure and abbreviations such as *OD*.

Operation: Removal of 3-cm nevus, lateral aspect, right knee.
Diagnosis: Cataract, OD.

periods

Do not use periods within or after most abbreviations, including acronyms, abbreviated units of measure, and brief forms. Periods must be used with abbreviated English units of measure if they may be misread without the period. It is preferable to write out most English units of measure, so it is easy to avoid this inconsistent use of the period in their abbreviated forms.

inch *preferred to* in. *Do not use* in *(without a period).*
mg
prep
WBC
wbc
exam

Do use periods in lowercased drug-related abbreviations.

b.i.d.
q.4h.
p.o.
p.r.n.

Do not use periods with abbreviated degrees and professional credentials.

BA
CMT

The use of periods with courtesy titles (e.g., Mr., Ms.) and following *Jr.* and *Sr.* varies.

If a sentence terminates with an abbreviation that requires a period, do not add another period.

He takes Valium 5 mg q.a.m.
not He takes Valium 5 mg q.a.m..

plurals
Use a lowercased *s* without an apostrophe to form the plural of capitalized abbreviations.

WBCs
EEGs
PVCs

Use *'s* to form the plural of lowercased abbreviations.

rbc's

possession
In general, add *'s* to show possession.

The AMA's address is ...

unusual abbreviations
Some abbreviations do not follow the usual pattern of all capitals. Learn the most common exceptions, and consult appropriate references for guidance.

pH
aVL
PhD
RPh

with numerals
Do not separate a numeral from its associated unit of measure or accompanying abbreviation. Specifically, do not allow a numeral to appear at the end of one line of type and its accompanying unit of measure or abbreviation at the beginning of the next line (or vice versa). Place both on the same line.

..................................The specimen measured 4 cm
in diameter.

or

................................The specimen measured
4 cm in diameter.

not

................................The specimen measured 4
cm in diameter.

See specific entries, including
acronyms
ampersand
Appendix CC, "State Names and Abbreviations, Major Cities, and
    State/City Resident Designations"
blank
brief forms
business names
chemical nomenclature
credentials, professional
degrees, academic
diagnoses
drug terminology
genus and species names
geographic names
International System of Measuring Units
Latin abbreviations
obstetrics terminology
personal names, nicknames, and initials
state, county, city, and town names and resident designations
time
titles
units of measure
USPS guidelines

-able, -ible

There is no shortcut to determining whether a term ends in *-able* or
-ible. Consult appropriate references for guidance.

abort, abortion, aborta

See obstetrics terminology

a.c.
    See drug terminology

academic degrees
    See degrees, academic

accent marks
    Also known as diacritics or diacritical marks, accent marks indicate pronunciation. Those that may be encountered in medical transcription include the following.

accent	*example*
acute	Calvé-Perthes disease
cedilla	François Chaussier sign
circumflex	bête rouge
dieresis	naïve
grave	boutonnière deformity
ring	Ångstrom
tilde	jalapeño
umlaut	Grüntzig catheter
virgule	Brønsted acid

    Many words once spelled with accents no longer require them, e.g., resume, facade, cooperation, naive, fiancee.

    The current trend is toward omitting accents in medical transcription because of equipment limitations and the likelihood of error when using them.

    Use of accents is required only rarely, such as in proper names, but omit them if the equipment cannot provide them.

    Never enter accent marks by hand.

    When you use accent marks, check appropriate references to determine accurate usage.

acceptable alternative forms
    See
    alternative acceptable forms
    "Introduction"

acronyms

Acronyms, also known as initialisms, are abbreviations formed with the initial letters of each of the successive parts or major parts of a compound term or of selected letters of the word or phrase. Some are pronounceable as words.

AAMT
laser
GI
IV

Clarity of communication is essential. Avoid the use of acronyms except for internationally recognized and accepted units of measure and for widely recognized terms and symbols. Do not use acronyms that readers will not readily recognize. Do not reduce unfamiliar terms to acronyms.

Unless the acronym is so widely used that it has in essence become a term in its own right, use the expanded term first, followed by its acronym in parentheses. Then use the acronym throughout the remainder of the document.

business / organization acronyms

For acronyms representing businesses and organizations, follow the style preference of the business or organization.

AAMT   American Association for Medical Transcription
NOCA   National Organization for Competency Assurance

capitalization

Capitalize all letters of most acronyms, but do not capitalize the words from which they are formed unless they are proper names.

AIDS (**a**cquired **i**mmuno**d**eficiency **s**yndrome)
TURP (**t**rans**u**rethral **r**esection of **p**rostate)
PERRLA (**p**upils **e**qual, **r**ound, **r**eactive to **l**ight and **a**ccommodation)

Most acronyms that have become words in their own right are lowercased. Many users of these terms are not aware that such terms are acronyms and do not know what terms the letters represent.

laser (**l**ight **a**mplification by **s**timulated **e**mission of **r**adiation)

Check appropriate references to determine current preferred forms and usage.

periods
Do not use periods with acronyms; they are old-fashioned and interfere with pronunciation. Exception: Occasionally, an entity will use periods in its own acronym; follow its preference.

plurals
Use *'s* to form the plural of lowercased acronyms. Use a lowercased *s* without an apostrophe to form the plural of capitalized acronyms.

WBCs
wbc's

possession
In general, add *'s* to show possession.

The AMA's address is ...

terms dictated as acronyms
Either use the acronym or transcribe the term in full when the acronym form is dictated. Exception: Abbreviations, including acronyms, are not acceptable in sections of reports giving names of diagnoses or operations.
Note: Throughout the text, the abbreviations D *and* T *have been used to indicate* dictated *and* transcribed, *respectively.*

D: The patient reported history of CABG.
T: The patient reported history of CABG.
or The patient reported history of coronary artery bypass graft.

but
D: Operation: CABG.
T: Operation: Coronary artery bypass graft.

terms dictated in full
Do not use acronyms when the terms they represent are dictated in full rather than in acronym form.

The patient reported history of coronary artery bypass graft.
(not *CABG*, unless dictated *cabbage* or the letters *CABG*)

uncertain meaning
If you cannot determine the meaning of the dictated acronym, either because it is unfamiliar to you or because it could have more than one meaning, transcribe the acronym, then flag the report requesting that the dictator extend the acronym and let you know its meaning for your future reference.

See
abbreviations
business names

acting (as part of a title)
Capitalize only when part of a capitalized title.

Charles Woodward, acting president
Acting-President Woodward

See titles

acute accent mark (´)
See accent marks

addresses

commas
Use commas to separate the parts of an address in narrative form. Exception: Do not place a comma before the ZIP code.

The patient's address is 139 Goddard Street, Modesto, CA 95355.

numbers
Always use figures (even number 1) to refer to house numbers. Do not use commas.

1 Eighth Avenue
1408 51st Street
101st Street
14084 Albany Avenue

No. or # may be used before an apartment, suite, or room number. Do not use before a house number.

1408 Albany Avenue, Apt. #148

See
street names and numbers
USPS guidelines

address requirements, post office
See USPS guidelines

When you catch an adjective, kill it.
Mark Twain

adjectives
Adjectives modify nouns and sometimes pronouns. The abbreviation *adj* is used in this book where it is necessary to identify adjectival forms.
Use commas to separate two or more adjectives if each modifies the noun alone. Do not place a comma between the last adjective and the modified noun.

Physical exam reveals a pleasant, cooperative, elderly female in
no acute distress.
The abdomen is soft, nontender, and supple.

If an adjective modifies a combination of the following adjective(s) and noun, do not use a comma to separate the adjectives.

This 54-year-old Caucasian female was referred to my office for
evaluation.
She did not have audible paroxysmal tachycardia.

Use commas to set off an adjective or adjectival phrase directly following the noun it modifies.

Diagnosis: Fracture, left tibia.
He has degenerative arthritis, left knee, with increasing inability
    to cope.
Blood cultures, all of which were negative, were drawn at four-hour
    intervals.

Some adjectives are identical to adverbs.

adj	*adv*
hard work	play *hard*
light color	travel *light*

See
compound modifiers
incomparable words

adnexa

Adnexa is always plural in usage.

The adnexa are normal.
Left adnexa are normal.
Left and right adnexa are normal.

adolescent

See age referents

adult

See age referents

adverbs

Adverbs modify verbs, adjectives, and other adverbs. The abbreviation
adv is used in this book where it is necessary to identify adverbial forms.
Some but not all adverbs end in *-ly*.

sterilely

Some adverbs are identical to adjectives.

adv   *adj*
play *hard*   *hard* work
travel *light*   *light* color

When an adverb is used with a compound verb, it may be placed between the parts of the verb, provided such placement does not obstruct the meaning.

He will routinely return for followup.

Traditionalists do not split an infinitive verb form with an adverb, but it is increasingly acceptable to do so. Transcribe as dictated, provided the phrasing does not obstruct the meaning.

The test was intended to definitively determine the diagnosis.

conjunctive adverbs
   See *conjunctions*

squinting modifiers
   A squinting modifier is an adverb that is placed in such a way that it can be interpreted as modifying more than one word. If the intended meaning can be determined, recast the sentence so that the modifier clearly relates to the appropriate word. See how the placement of *only* in the following sentence changes the meaning.

   He only walked two blocks. *(he only walked, not ran)*
   Only he walked two blocks. *(only he, not anyone else, walked two blocks)*
   He walked only two blocks. *(he didn't walk more than two blocks)*

   So the squinting modifier *only* in "He only walked two blocks" should be moved so that the sentence reads "He walked only two blocks."

   See
   compound modifiers
   however

affect, effect
   These terms often sound alike in pronunciation, but their usage and meanings are not interchangeable.

What you and I need is the right word—
fat or thin, brisk or lazy. The right word.
In the right place. For the right reason.
Willard R. Espy

affect
A verb meaning to influence; a noun meaning an expressed or observed emotion or feeling.

The treatment affected the symptoms.
The patient displayed a flat affect.

effect
A verb meaning to bring about; a noun meaning result.

The medication effected relief.
The effect of the treatment was pronounced.

African-American, African American
See sociocultural designations

age referents

neonates and newborns
Children from birth to 1 month of age. Refer to them also as boys and girls and children.

infants
Children from 1 month to 24 months (2 years) of age. Refer to them also as boys and girls and children.

child, children
Boys and girls aged 2 to 13 years. These terms may also be used for those from birth to 13 years. Refer to them also as boys and girls.

adolescents, youths, teenagers
Boys and girls aged 13 through 17 years. Refer to them also as boys and girls.

boys and girls
Neonates, children and adolescents, i.e., people from birth through 17 years. Refer to them also as neonates, newborns, children, adolescents, youths, and teenagers, depending on their age.

adults
People aged 18 years or older. Refer to them also as men and women.

man, men; woman, women
Adults, i.e., people aged 18 years or older. Refer to them also as adults.

See
ages
sexist language

Adolescence is schizophrenia with a good prognosis.
Thomas L. Coleman

ages
Use numerals to express ages, except at the beginning of a sentence.

7-year-old patient
3½-year-old child

at the beginning of sentence
Recast the sentence or write out the number.

D: 7-year-old patient who …
T: A 7-year-old patient who …
or Seven-year-old patient who …

as adjectives before nouns or as noun substitutes
Use hyphens. Do not use hyphens if the phrase does not precede the noun.

15-year-old boy *not* 15 year old boy
13-year-olds *not* 13 year olds
The patient, who is 15 years old ...

> ### The hardest years in life are those between ten and seventy.
> Helen Hayes

In phrases where the noun following the verb is implied, hyphens are used. Alternatively, edit to a form that does not require hyphens.

The patient, a 3-year-old, was not yet walking. (The word *patient* is implied following *3-year-old*)
or The patient, 3 years old, was not yet walking.

decade references
Use numerals. Do not use an apostrophe.

The patient is in her 50s. (*not* 50's, *not* fifties)

See
age referents
fractions
numbers

agreement, subject-verb
See verb-subject agreement

a.k.a.
Abbreviation meaning *also known as*. Use lowercased letters with periods to distinguish from *AKA*, meaning above-knee amputation.

Muhammed Ali, a.k.a. Cassius Clay, was admitted to the hospital.

alfa
Variant spelling for *alpha,* used especially in generic drug names. Check references for applications.

- alfa interferon

See drug terminology

alleles
See genetics terminology

allergies
Some institutions use capitals or bold type to draw attention to a patient's allergies. Regular type is, of course, also acceptable. Do not underline or use italics; either reduces readability.

ALLERGIES: penicillin and aspirin.
or ALLERGIES: PENICILLIN AND ASPIRIN.
or **ALLERGIES**: penicillin and aspirin.
or **ALLERGIES: penicillin and aspirin.**
but not ALLERGIES: penicillin and aspirin.
and not *ALLERGIES: penicillin and aspirin.*

almost never
Avoid. Edit to *seldom* or *hardly ever.*

D: He almost never arrives on time.
T: He hardly ever arrives on time.

alphanumeric terms
Terms composed of letters and numerals; they may include symbols. Rules vary. Check appropriate headings and references for guidance.

L4-5
T4
3M

alternate, alternative
Soundalikes, not synonyms. Beware of misuse.

alternate
Taking turns in succession (adj), occurring in turns (v), a substitute (n).

Valium was given in alternate doses of 5 mg and 10 mg.

alternative
Choice.

The alternatives were chemotherapy or radiation therapy.

alternative acceptable forms
Different transcription styles and practices that are acceptable but not necessarily preferred. AAMT attempts to present the most preferred forms, acknowledging equally (or almost equally) acceptable forms, but we do not attempt to present all acceptable forms.
It is important to note that even forms that are widely used and/or well documented may not be correct, e.g., *Verres* needle continues to be both widely used and documented, but the correct form is *Veress*. Thus, AAMT would not acknowledge *Verres* as an alternative acceptable form.

See
"Introduction"
spelling

although, though

although
A subordinating conjunction that joins a dependent clause to a main clause.
When the *although* clause precedes the main clause, it is usually followed by a comma. When it follows the main clause, it may be preceded by a comma if the comma assists clarity and understanding; the comma may be omitted if its omission does not confuse the reader.

Although he was frightened, the child cooperated fully with the exam.
The child cooperated fully with the exam although he was frightened.
or
The child cooperated fully with the exam, although he was frightened.

though
An adverb. It is not necessary to set it off by commas unless there is
a break in continuity or a need for a pause in reading.

It was difficult for him. He did it though.

a.m., AM; p.m., PM
Acceptable abbreviations for *ante meridiem* and *post meridiem*.

a.m., p.m.
Preferred forms. Use periods (so *a.m.* won't be misread as the word
am). Precede and follow *a.m.* or *p.m.* by a space.

4 a.m.
5:30 p.m.

AM, PM
Acceptable but not preferred because the capitals draw more atten-
tion to themselves than to the time. When used, do not use periods.
Precede and follow *AM* or *PM* by a space.

4 AM
5:30 PM

redundant phrases
Do not accompany *a.m.* and *p.m.* expressions with redundant phrases
such as *in the morning, in the evening, tonight, o'clock.*

8:15 a.m. *not* 8:15 a.m. o'clock
10:30 a.m. *not* 10:30 a.m. in the morning

See time

American Association for Medical Transcription (AAMT)

National professional association for medical transcriptionists, with members throughout the United States and in several other countries. Abbreviation: AAMT (no periods).

AAMT's mission is the advancement of medical transcription and the education and development of medical transcriptionists as medical language specialists. It carries out this mission by:

- Being a leader in the development and advancement of medical transcription standards, ethics, and curriculum.

- Representing and promoting the interests of medical transcription and medical language specialists.

- Shaping and promoting the education of medical language specialists.

- Encouraging and assisting the professional development of medical language specialists.

- Participating in the development and advancement of technologies related to the practice of medical transcription.

- Advocating the medical language specialist as a communications and documentation partner in the assurance of quality patient care.

- Representing the medical transcription profession in public and private initiatives to improve quality patient care documentation.

- Serving as the primary source for information related to medical transcription.

Founded in 1978 as a not-for-profit corporation, AAMT is led by a nine-member board of directors elected by active members and a house of delegates (including the AAMT board of directors and delegates from recognized state/regional associations). It is managed by staff at its administrative office in Modesto, California.

Membership categories include active (medical transcriptionists), as well as associate, student, institutional, and corporate, and there is a Business Issues Section for business owners.

Nearly 200 local chapters and state/regional associations are located throughout the United States and in Canada. AAMT assists in the formation and operation of these component associations through publications, a board-liaison program, on-site visits, leadership programs and publications, and telephone communications.

The association publishes a bimonthly journal (*JAAMT*) for all members, a bimonthly newsletter for component association leaders, and educational, informational, and promotional materials, including position papers, press releases, videos, modules (transcription tapes and transcripts), model curriculum, model job description, and humor books.

Education programs include an annual meeting, as well as annual conferences on business, education, leadership, and supervision/management.

The association also administers a professional certification program, the *Medical Transcriptionist Certification Program at AAMT*.

For more information on the association and its programs, products, and services, contact its administrative office:

AAMT
PO Box 576187
Modesto, CA 95357-6187

Telephone: 800-982-2182 or 209-551-0883
Fax: 209-551-9317

See
AAMT
Medical Transcriptionist Certification Program at AAMT

amino acids
See genetics terminology

amount of
Takes a singular verb.

A minimal amount of bleeding was present.
The amount of adhesions was minimal.

ampersand (&)
Symbol meaning *and*. Do not use except in special instances.

---

in abbreviations

Use with certain single-letter abbreviations separated by *and*. Do not space before or after the ampersand. Check appropriate references to identify acceptable uses. Do not use ampersand forms in operative titles or diagnoses.

D&C
T&A

D: Operation: D&C.
T: Operation: Dilatation and curettage.

See business names

an

See
a, an
articles

anatomic terms

features

Do not capitalize the names of anatomic features (except the eponyms associated with them).

ligament of Treitz
os frontale
zygomatic bone

posture-based terms

anterior	nearer the front
posterior	nearer the rear
superior	nearer the top
inferior	nearer the bottom

region-based terms

cranial, cephalic	nearer the head
caudal	nearer the tail end
dorsal	nearer the back
ventral	nearer the belly side

directional and positional terms

Form directional adverbs by replacing the adjectival suffix (*-al, -or, -ic*) with the suffix *-ad,* meaning *-ward.* Use these forms in the same type of constructions in which *-ward* forms are used.

    caudad
    cephalad
    craniad
    laterad
    orad
    superiad
    ventrad

Do not substitute the *-ad* form when the *-ly* adverb or the adjective itself has been used correctly.

    the anterior incision
    It extends caudally from ...

Use a combining vowel to join directional and positional adjectives.

    mediolateral

Latin and English names

It is common practice for dictators to mix the English and Latin names of anatomic parts, i.e., using English for the noun and Latin for the adjectives. These may be transcribed as dictated or edited to either their English or Latin forms.

    latissimus dorsi muscle
    peroneus profundus nerve
    palbebrales arteries
    temporales profundi veins
    transverse abdominis muscle

and/or

Dictated "and or." Used to indicate that one or the other or both of the items connected to it are involved. Note that a virgule is placed between the two words; do not hyphenate.

    We are considering surgery and/or chemotherapy.

and others

Latin equivalent is *et al.*

See Latin abbreviations

and so forth

Latin equivalent is *et cetera,* abbreviated *etc.* Do not use *and so forth* (or its Latin equivalent) when the list is preceded by *e.g.,* or *for example.*

See Latin abbreviations

angles

In expressing angles, write out *degrees* in text. Use degree sign (°) only in tables.

Flexion to 40 degrees.
not Flexion to 40°.

See degrees

ante meridiem

See a.m., AM; p.m., PM

APGAR questionnaire

Acronym from initial letters of *adaptability, partnership, growth, affection, resolve,* referring to a family assessment instrument. Use all capitals. Do not confuse with Apgar score.

See scores

Apgar score

See scores

apostrophes

Apostrophes have many uses, the most common being to show possession, to form some plurals, and to denote omitted letters or numbers in contractions. Knowing when not to use apostrophes is as important as knowing when to use them. Medical transcription rules for apostrophes generally reflect those of common usage. Be sure to use the appropriate symbol for the apostrophe ('), if available, instead of the prime sign (').

See specific topic entries for related guidelines, as well as
contractions
plurals
possession

appositives
Words or phrases before or after a noun that explain or identify it.

essential appositives
Do not use commas to set off essential appositives (those essential to the meaning of the sentence).

Her brother Walter was tested as a potential bone marrow donor. *(Patient has more than one brother so must specify which is being referenced.)*

nonessential appositives
Use a comma before and after nonessential appositives (those not essential to the meaning of the sentence).

The surgeons, Dr. Jones and Dr. Smith, reported that the procedure was a success.

April
See months

arabic numerals
See
International System of Measuring Units
numbers
units of measure

area
See International System of Measuring Units

area code

See telephone numbers

army, Army

Capitalize when referring to US Army, lowercase when referring to other nations' armies and for generic references.

The patient is a private in the US Army.
The patient is a private in the Israeli army.
They are scheduled for army physicals.

articles

The articles *a, an,* and *the* are modifiers that are used to indicate definiteness (*the*) or indefiniteness (*a, an*) of the noun that follows. Articles are frequently dropped in dictation. They may be transcribed or not (whether dictated or not) provided their presence or absence does not substantially change the meaning or style of the dictator. Articles are more apt to be included in correspondence than in reports. When dropped in transcription, it is usually because they were not dictated, they were not heard by the transcriptionist, or they were not dictated elsewhere in the report and the transcriptionist is seeking some consistency.

with abbreviations

The use of articles with abbreviations varies. Sometimes the article is required. Sometimes it is optional. Sometimes it should not be used.

required

We will do a CBC.

optional

She was admitted to the ICU.
or She was admitted to ICU.

omission required

AAMT is ...
not The AAMT is ...
but The American Association for Medical Transcription is ...

See
a, an
the

as

Use *as,* not *like,* as a conjunction to introduce clauses.

He took the medication *as* he was instructed.
not He took the medication *like* he was instructed.

as if, as though

Both acceptable but *as if* is preferred. Transcribe as dictated.

as to

Acceptable when dictated at the beginning of a sentence, but when used elsewhere, remove it or replace it by a single word, e.g., *why, about, in.*

As to the lab results ...

D: She inquired as to the reasons for the procedure.
T: She inquired about the reasons for the procedure.

D: Her concerns as to the prognosis ...
T: Her concerns regarding the prognosis ...

See like

assistant, associate

Do not abbreviate. Capitalize only when part of a formal title before a name, but such use is rare because the terms usually represent job or occupational titles, not formal titles (even when placed before a name). Use appositional construction wherever possible.

The assistant surgeon, Dr. Jones, closed the wound.
Dr. Jones, the assistant surgeon, closed the wound.

See
appositives
titles

associations

See business names

at large

Do not hyphenate the noun form.

members at large
delegates at large

Hyphenate the adjective form.

members-at-large meeting
delegates-at-large assembly

audit trails

Also known as documentation trails, audit trails contribute to risk management. An audit trail is simply a careful sequential record of actions and conversations on a matter. They are recommended for any particularly legally sensitive event, including circumstances where medical transcriptionists are advised or directed to act contrary to appropriate practices or legal directives.

See
Appendix B, "The Mark of Zorro"
Appendix C, "When Did 'CMT' Become 'MD'?"
date dictated, date transcribed
dictated but not read
professional liability insurance
risk management
transcribed but not read
verbatim transcription

August

See months

authentication

The process of (a) proving authorship, for example, by written signature, identifiable initials, or computer key, and (b) proving that a document is what it purports to be, such as by comparison with other records.

See
Appendix C, "When Did 'CMT' Become 'MD'?"

Appendix D, "What's Wrong With This Picture?"
Appendix E, "AAMT Position Paper: Providers' Signatures"
dictated but not read
risk management
transcribed but not read

author
One who creates the document, whether it be a report, letter, manuscript, or other and whether it is by dictation or other means. Also called dictator or originator.

See authentication

autoauthentication
See Appendix D, "What's Wrong With This Picture?"

automobiles
Capitalize brand names, but lowercase generic terms.

Ford Taurus
Honda Civic
Oldsmobile sedan
Chevrolet station wagon

autopsy report
Report prepared by a pathologist or medical examiner to document findings on examination of cadaver. Typical content topics include:

medical history
course of treatment
external exam or description
evidence of injury
macroscopic exam
internal exam
gross findings (systems and organs)
special dissections and examinations
microscopic exam
findings
opinion

pathologic diagnosis
cause of death

See formats

autumn
See seasons

average of
Takes a plural verb if preceded by *an,* singular if preceded by *the.*

An average of 10 tests were done on each patient.
The average of the results was 48.3%.

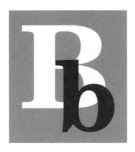

B cells, B lymphocytes
See lymphocyte and monoclonal antibody nomenclature

BA, AB
Abbreviations for *Bachelor of Arts* degree.

See
bachelor's degree
degrees, academic

bachelor's degree
Lowercase this generic form, but use capitals when the specific form or abbreviation is used, e.g., Bachelor of Arts (BA) degree or Bachelor of Science (BS) degree.

See degrees, academic

back-formations
Verbs formed from nouns; a form of coined term. They are frequently encountered in medical dictation. Use dictated back-formations only if they have become acceptable through widespread use. Avoid other back-formations.

Do not capitalize a back-formation derived from a capitalized noun, e.g., a brand name or eponym.

back-formation	*noun form*
to diagnose	diagnosis
to dialyze	dialysis

to biopsy	biopsy
to dehisce	dehiscence
to bovie	Bovie
to heparinize	heparin
to digitalize	digitalis

We will dialyze the patient tomorrow.
The wound was dehisced.

Some back-formations that have been attempted but are unlikely to become accepted include *prophylaxed* (from *prophylaxis*), *life flighted* (from *Life Flight*), and *guaiaced* (from *guaiac*).

See
coined terms
editing

> ***The English language has far more lives than a cat. People have been murdering it for years.***
> Farmers' Almanac

Ballard scale
See scales

basic 4 reports
The basic 4 reports are consultation report, discharge summary, history and physical examination, and operative report.

See
Appendix A, "Sample Reports"
consultation report
discharge summary
formats
history and physical examination
operative report

basic fundamental

The two words have the same meaning, so the phrase is redundant.
Use one or the other.

The basic problem was ...
or The fundamental problem was ...
not The basic fundamental problem was ...

bastard enumeration

Also known as unparallel series.

See series

bay

Capitalize when integral part of a proper name and in popular names
that are widely used and accepted; otherwise, lowercase.

Morro Bay
San Francisco Bay
the Bay Area
He walked along the bay.

bc

Abbreviation for *blind copy.*

See copy designation

beats per minute

Spell out; do not abbreviate.

Pulse: 70 beats per minutes.
not Pulse: 70 bpm.

Why shouldn't we quarrel about a word?
What is the good of words if they aren't
important enough to quarrel over?
Why do we choose one word more than another
if there isn't any difference between them?
G.K. Chesterton

because, due to, since

because
> Denotes a specific cause-effect relationship.
>
> He has been in pain because his arm was broken.

due to
> Means caused by or resulting from, not *because*.
>
> Her reaction was due to a penicillin allergy.
> *not* Her reaction was because of a penicillin allergy.
>
> She was late because her watch stopped.
> *not* She was late due to her watch stopping.

since
> Indicates an event follows another but was not caused by it.
>
> He has been in pain since he returned from vacation.

before, prior to
> Use *before* instead of *prior to* except when a sense of requirement is intended.
>
> He was seen in the emergency room before admission.
> *but* He must pay the fee prior to admission.

Berkow formula
See classifications

biannual, biennial, bimonthly, biweekly

biannual
A *biannual* event happens twice yearly. Synonym: semiannual.

biennial
A *biennial* event happens every two years.

bimonthly
A bimonthly event occurs every two months. Do not confuse with *semimonthly,* meaning twice monthly.

biweekly
A biweekly event occurs every two weeks. Do not confuse with *semiweekly,* meaning twice weekly.

See semiannual, semimonthly, semiweekly

b.i.d.
See drug terminology

bilateral
Adjective that may modify a singular or plural noun, depending on meaning.

A bilateral decision ...
Diagnosis: Bilateral pneumonia.
Operation: Bilateral mastectomies.

biochemical terminology
See
chemical nomenclature
genetics terminology

biopsy

The back-formation of the noun *biopsy* into a verb form is common in medical dictation, so transcribe it as dictated.

The liver was biopsied.
or A biopsy of the liver was done.

See back-formations

birthday

Capitalize only when part of the name of an official holiday; otherwise, lowercase.

Lincoln's Birthday
He was injured at his birthday party.

black, Black

See sociocultural designations

blank

When a dictated abbreviation, term, or phrase is indecipherable, unrecognizable, or cannot be confirmed through reasonable research, leave a blank and flag the report, briefly explaining why you left a blank, noting what the dictation sounds like, and asking for feedback for future reference. **Never** make it appear that a transcript is complete by "closing up" the space where the indecipherable or difficult word, phrase, or sentence belongs. Appropriate use of blanks and the followup they should prompt contribute to clinical care and risk management.

See
editing
errors in dictation
flag
risk management

blind copy

See copy designation

blood counts

differential blood count
Part of a white blood cell count. Includes polymorphonuclear neutrophils (PMNs, polys, segmented neutrophils [segs]), band neutrophils (bands, stabs), lymphocytes (lymphs), eosinophils (eos), basophils (basos), and monocytes (monos). Counts may be given as whole numbers or as percents; total should equal 100 in either case.

White blood count of 4800, with 58% segs, 7% bands, 24% lymphs, 8% monos, 1% eos, and 2% basos.
or White blood count of 4800, with 58 segs, 7 bands, 24 lymphs, 8 monos, 1 eo, and 2 basos.

RBC, rbc
RBC is preferred abbreviation for red blood count; *rbc,* for red blood cells.

WBC, wbc
WBC is preferred abbreviation for white blood count; *wbc,* for white blood cells.

white blood count
See differential blood count *above.*

blood groups

ABO system
Use single or dual letters, sometimes with a subscript letter or number. Where subscripts are not possible, place the numeral immediately following and on-line with the letter.

group A
group A_1 *or* group A1
group AB
group A_1B *or* group A1B

Other common blood group systems include Auberger, Diego, Duffy, Kell, Kidd, Lewis, Lutheran, Rh (not *Rhesus*), Sutter, and Xg. Consult appropriate references for guidance in expressing terms related to these and other blood groups.

blood pressure (BP)

Reported in *mmHg* (or *mm Hg*), but sometimes just the values are dictated.

Do not delete *mmHg* if dictated, but it may be added if not dictated. Use abbreviation *BP* if dictated; otherwise, use extended form.

D: BP 110/80
T: BP 110/80 *or* BP 110/80 mmHg *or* blood pressure 110/80

body cavities

Body spaces that contain internal organs.

cavity	organs
cranial	brain
thoracic	esophagus, trachea, thymus gland, aorta, lungs, heart
abdominal	gallbladder, liver, spleen, pancreas, stomach, small intestine, large intestine
pelvic	urinary bladder, urethra, ureters (in female: uterus and vagina, as well)
spinal	nerves of spinal cord

body parts

Phrases such as *left heart* and *right chest* are frequently dictated when what is meant is *left side of heart, right side of chest*. These phrases may be transcribed as dictated unless their usage would confuse or amuse rather than communicate.

left heart catheterization
right lung abscess
left neck incision

bold type

In general, avoid bold type in medical transcription. A common exception is the use of bold type to designate a patient's allergies, although regular type is also acceptable.

ALLERGIES: Penicillin.

See
allergies
regular type

boy
See age referents

braces ({})
See
chemical nomenclature
parentheses

brackets ([])
See
chemical nomenclature
parentheses

brain death
See Harvard criteria for brain death

brand name
See names

breaths per minute
See pulmonary and respiratory terms

brief forms
Shortened forms of words. These may be transcribed as dictated if they are commonly used and widely recognized, but they should be extended in headings, diagnoses, and operative titles.
Lowercase brief forms unless the extended form should be capitalized. Do not use an ending period. Form the plural by adding *s* (no apostrophe) to the term itself or the accompanying noun if the term is used as an adjective.

phones	telephones
exams	examinations
Pap smears	Papanicolaou smears

See abbreviations

bring, take

Use *bring* to signify movement toward. Use *take* to signify movement away from.

She will bring in a urine specimen on her next visit.
She took the urine specimen to the laboratory.

British spelling

Some terms are spelled differently in the United States than in Great Britain. Use the form that is preferred in the country in which you are transcribing. Note: British forms may also be Canadian forms.

British:	paediatric, orthopaedic, aluminium, metre, honour
US:	pediatric, orthopedic, aluminum, meter, honor

British thermal unit (BTU)

Use abbreviation (BTU) with arabic numerals. Use same form for singular or plural.

1 BTU
4 BTU

Broders index

See cancer classifications

Brown and Sharp gauge

System for sizing sutures. Abbreviation: B&S gauge.

See suture sizes

bruit
>	*See* cardiology terminology

BS
>	Abbreviation for *Bachelor of Science* degree.
>
>	*See*
>	bachelor's degree
>	degrees, academic

BTU
>	*See* British thermal unit (BTU)

building, structure, and room names
>	Capitalize proper names of office buildings, government buildings, churches, hospitals, hotels. Do not abbreviate. Capitalize the word *building* only if it is an integral part of the official name.
>
>	the White House
>	Memorial Hospital
>	Empire State Building
>	*but* the Damrell building
>
>	Capitalize proper names of structures, monuments, etc. Lowercase generic terms.
>
>	She fell while visiting the Tomb of the Unknown Soldier.
>	He tripped on the steps of the Capitol.
>	She fell against the Rodin sculpture.
>
>	Do not capitalize common nouns designating rooms; these are generic terms applied to all similar rooms. Capitalize names of specially designated rooms only.
>
>	He was admitted through the emergency room.
>	She left the operating room in good condition.
>	She fell at a reception in the Rose Room.
>
>	Use abbreviations for room names only if dictated **and** if they will be readily recognized by the reader.

He was admitted to the ICU.
or He was admitted to the intensive care unit.

Use arabic numerals for room numbers. Lowercase *room*.

The patient is in room 148.

See
business names
names
nouns

bur, burr
The preferred medical spelling is *bur*.

burn classifications
See classifications

business names
Express according to the business's style and usage. Except for businesses that are as well known by their abbreviations as by their full names (IBM, for example), use the full name before using the abbreviated form in order to avoid confusion among similar abbreviations.

In general, capitalize complete names (except articles and prepositions). Note: If the entity uses lowercase, do likewise.

American Association for Medical Transcription (AAMT)
Computer-based Patient Record Institute (CPRI)
American Medical Association (AMA)
American Management Association (AMA)

Capitalize words such as *organization, institution, association* only when part of the entity's official name; do not capitalize them when they are used alone or in a shortened version of the name. Note: The entity, in shortened references to itself, may choose to use initial capitals.

American Hospital Association *but* the association *or* the hospital
association
American Association for Medical Transcription *or* the association *or*
the Association *(in references to itself)*

abbreviations / acronyms

Some businesses are readily recognized by their abbreviations or acronyms and may be referred to by same if dictated and if there is reasonable assurance the business will be accurately identified by the reader. Most abbreviated forms use all capitals and do not use periods, but be guided by the entity's designated abbreviated form. For example, *AAMT* is the preferred form for the American Association for Medical Transcription—all capitals, no periods.

IBM equipment
He is an ACLU attorney.

ampersand

Use an ampersand (&) in company, corporation, partnership names when it is part of that entity's formal expression of its name. In these instances, space before and after the ampersand if it separates words or multiple letters; do not space if it separates single letters.

Bausch & Lomb
S&H

company, Company

Capitalize *company* only if part of an official name.

Campbell Soup Company
company policy

Co., Corp., Inc., Ltd.

Abbreviate and capitalize *Co., Corp., Inc.,* or *Ltd.* only when the business being named uses the abbreviation in its formal name. Do not use a comma before *Inc.* or *Ltd.* unless the specific entity chooses to use it.

Ford Motor Co.

Retain capitalization of other terms if *Co., Corp., Inc.,* or *Ltd.,* is deleted.

American Association of Medical Assistants, Inc.
or American Association of Medical Assistants

Form possessive of names using abbreviation *Co., Corp., Inc.,* or *Ltd.* as follows.

Ford Motor Co.'s annual report

departments
Lowercase common nouns designating department names, reserving capitals for proper nouns or adjectives, in addresses, or when part of a federal government agency name. Use abbreviations for departments only if dictated **and** if they will be readily recognized by the reader.

the surgery department of St. Mary's Hospital
Mount St. Mary's emergency room

The letter was addressed as follows:
Chief, Emergency Department
Mount Zion Hospital
San Francisco, CA 95351

He works for the State Department in Washington, DC.
She is head of the surgery department.
He is head of ICU.
The patient is head of the English department at the local state
    university.

divisions
Lowercase common nouns naming institutional divisions.

The administrative division of Memorial Hospital ...

internal units
Lowercase common names for internal units of an organization. Exception: Capitalization may be used for such internal units in the entity's references to itself in its own formal and/or legal documents.

the board of directors of AAMT
AAMT board of directors *(except perhaps* AAMT Board of Directors
    in formal and / or legal documents)

Capitalize internal elements when their names are not generic terms.

the Business Issues Section of AAMT

inverted forms
When inverted forms of names are widely used and recognized, capitalize those forms as well.

College of William and Mary
William and Mary College

See
abbreviations
building, structure, and room names
names
nouns

businessperson(s)
Preferred to *businessman / businessmen, businesswoman / business-woman*.

See sexist language

but* meaning *only
When *but* is used to mean *only*, it is a negative and should not be preceded by *not*.

D: She was not seen but once.
T: She was seen but once.

by (in dimensions)
Use a lowercased *x* to express *by* in dimensions. Space before and after the *x*.

13 x 2 cm

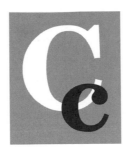

c, C, c̄

Abbreviation *c* is for *copy* and *C* is for *Celsius*.

The medical symbol c̄ meaning *with* is frequently used in handwritten notes. Use *with* in transcribed reports.

See
copy designation
temperature, temperature scales

caliber of weapons

Express with decimal point followed by arabic numerals and a hyphen. Do not place a zero before the decimal point.

.38-caliber pistol

Canada

Canadian spelling

Some terms are spelled differently in the United States than in Canada. Use the form that is preferred in the country in which you are transcribing. Note: Canadian forms may be the same as British forms.

Canadian: paediatric, orthopaedic, aluminium, metre, honour
US: pediatric, orthopedic, aluminum, meter, honor

Canadian territories and provinces

Capitalize full names of Canadian territories.

Northwest Territories

Yukon Territory

Use commas to set off community names from names of provinces. Do not capitalize *province*. Do not abbreviate names of provinces in reports.

She is from Toronto, Ontario. (*not* Toronto, Ont.)
the province of Ontario

French Canadian
Do not hyphenate.

See
geographic names
USPS guidelines

cancer classifications

stage and grade
Do not capitalize *stage* or *grade*. Use roman numerals for cancer stages, arabic numerals for grades. For subdivisions of cancer stages, add on-line capital letters and arabic suffixes, without spaces or hyphens.

stage 0
stage I   stage IA
stage II   stage II3
stage III
stage IV   stage IVB

grade 1
grade 2
grade 3
grade 4

Broders index
Classification of aggressiveness of tumor malignancy. Reported as grade 1 (most differentiation and best prognosis) through grade 4 (least differentiation and poorest diagnosis). Lowercase *grade,* use arabic numerals.

Broders grade 3

CIN grade
    CIN is an acronym for *cervical intraepithelial neoplasia.* Expressed
in grades from 1 through 3 (from least to greatest severity). Lowercase
grade, use arabic numerals, and place a hyphen between *CIN* and the
numeral.

    CIN-1
    CIN-2
    CIN-3

Clark level
    Describes invasion level of primary malignant melanoma of the skin
from the epidermis. Use roman numerals I (least deep) to IV (deepest).

Clark level I	into underlying papillary dermis
Clark level II	to junction of papillary and reticular dermis
Clark level III	into reticular dermis
Clark level IV	into the subcutaneous fat

Dukes classification
    Named for British pathologist Cuthbert E. Dukes (1890-1977).
Classifies extent of operable adenocarcinoma of the colon or rectum.
No apostrophe. Follow with capital letter.

Dukes A	confined to mucosa
Dukes B	extending into the muscularis mucosa
Dukes C	extending through the bowel wall, with metastasis to lymph nodes

FAB classification
    Acronym for **F**rench-**A**merican-**B**ritish. Morphologic classification
system for acute nonlymphoid leukemia. Express with capital *M* followed
by arabic numeral (1 through 6); do not space between the *M* and the
numeral.

M1	myeloblastic, no differentiation
M2	myeloblastic, differentiation
M3	promyelocytic
M4	myelomonocytic
M5	monocytic
M6	erythroleukemia

FAB staging of carcinoma utilizes TNM classification of malignant tumors. *See* TNM classification of malignant tumors *below.*

FAB T1, N1, M0

FIGO staging
Federation **I**nternationale de **G**ynécologie et **O**bstétrique's system for staging gynecologic malignancy, particularly carcinomas of the ovary. Expressed as stage I (least severe) to stage IV (most severe). Lowercase *stage,* and use roman numerals.

Diagnosis: Ovarian carcinoma, FIGO stage II.

Gleason tumor grade
Also known as Gleason score. The system scores or grades the prognosis for adenocarcinoma of prostate, with a scale of 1 through 5 for each dominant and secondary pattern, then totaled for score. The higher the score, the more severe the prognosis. Lowercase *grade* or *score,* and use arabic numerals.

Diagnosis: Adenocarcinoma of prostate, Gleason score 8.

Jewett classification of bladder carcinoma
Use capitals as follows:

O   in situ (note: letter *O,* not numeral *0*)
A   involving submucosa
B   involving muscle
C   involving surrounding tissue
D   involving distant sites

Diagnosis: Bladder carcinoma, Jewett class B.

Karnofsky rating scale, Karnofsky status
Scale for rating performance status of patients with malignant neoplasms. Use arabic numerals: 10, 20, 30, 40, 50, 60, 70, 80, 90, 100. (Normal is 100, moribund is 10.)

TNM classification of malignant tumors
System for staging malignant tumors, developed by the American Joint Committee on Cancer and the Union Internationale Contre le Cancer.

T   **tumor** size or involvement
N   regional lymph **node** involvement
M   extent of **metastasis**

Write TNM expressions with on-line arabic numerals and commas, spacing after the commas.

T2, N1, M1
T4, N3, M1

Letters and symbols following the letters T, N, and M:

X means assessment cannot be done.
0 indicates no evidence found.
Numbers indicate increasing evidence of the characteristics
    represented by those letters.
Tis indicates in situ tumor.

Tis, N0, M0

The TNM system criteria for defining cancer stages vary according to the type of cancer. Thus a stage II cancer of one type may be defined as T1, N0, M0, while one of another type may be defined as T2, N1, M0.
    Staging indicators are used along with TNM criteria to define cancers and assess stage. These are expressed with capital letters and arabic numerals.

grade	GX, G1, G2, G3
host performance	H0, H1, H2, H3, H4
lymphatic invasion	LX, L0, L1, L2
residual tumor	RX, R0, R1, R2
scleral invasion	S0, S0, S1, S2
venous invasion	VX, V0, V1, V2

Lowercased prefixes with TNM and other symbols indicate criteria used to describe and stage the tumor. Place the prefix on-line, e.g., cTNM, aT2.

letter	*determining criteria*
a	autopsy staging
c	clinical classification
p	pathological classification
r	retreatment classification
y, yp	classification during or following treatment with multiple modalities

cannot, can't

Use *cannot* instead of *can not* and *can't* except in direct quotations.

capitalization

Capitals emphasize and draw attention to the terms in which they are used. Their overuse can diminish their value and impact, so it is important to use them appropriately and judiciously.

Some words are always capitalized, some never. The placement or use of a term may determine whether it is capitalized; capitals, for example, are used to mark the beginning of a sentence.

Learning and adopting the rules of capitalization, when they should be used and when they should not be used, as well as the few instances when variations may be acceptable, will improve the consistency, accuracy, and communication value of transcribed medical reports.

In particular, avoid the use of unnecessary or inappropriate capitals. Do not, for example, capitalize a common-noun reference to a thing or person if it is just one of many other such things or persons. Thus, *emergency room* and *recovery room* are not capitalized. Think of the rule for generic versus brand names for drugs. The generic term (common noun) *emergency room* is applied to all emergency rooms, so it is not capitalized.

See specific entries for rules and guidelines, including:
abbreviations
acronyms
anatomic features
brief forms
building, structure, and room names
business names
cancer classifications
chemical nomenclature
classifications
credentials, professional
degrees, academic

disease names
drug terminology
formats
genus and species names
Greek letters
holidays and holy days
medical specialties
names
nouns
personal names, nicknames, and initials
quotations, quotation marks
scales
scores
seasons
sociocultural designations
state, county, city, and town names and resident designations
time zones
titles
units of measure
virus names
USPS guidelines

carbon copy
Copy of report or correspondence sent to someone other than addressee. Although *carbon* copy is now a misnomer, it is still widely used. Also known as *courtesy copy*. Abbreviation: cc (no periods).

See copy designation

cardiac murmur grades
See cardiology terminology

cardinal numbers
See numbers

cardiology terminology

electrocardiographic terms
ECG: Abbreviation for electrocardiogram, electrocardiography, electrocardiographic. Note: The use of *EKG* as an equivalent abbreviation is discouraged.

leads
Electronic connections for recording by means of electrocardiograph. Where subscripts are called for but not available, on-line standard-size numerals or letters may be used.

standard bipolar leads: Use roman numerals.

lead I, lead II, lead III

augmented limb leads: Lowercased *a* followed by a capital *V*, then a capital *R* (right), *L* (left), or *F* (front).

aVR, aVL, aVF.

precordial leads: Capital *V* followed by a subscript arabic numeral. If subscripting is not available, enter the numeral in the same point size on-line with the *V*, with no space between.

V_1, V_2, V_3, V_4, V_5, V_6, V_7, V_8, V_9
or V1, V2, V3, V4, V5, V6, V7, V8, V9

right precordial leads: Capital *V* followed by a subscript arabic numeral and subscript capital *R*. If subscripting is not available, enter the numeral and *R* in the same point size on-line with the *V*, with no space between.

V_{3R}, V_{4R}, etc.
or V3R, V4R, etc.

ensiform cartilage lead: Capital *V*, with subscript *E*. If subscripting is not available, enter *E* in the same point size on-line with the *V*, with no space between.

V_E *or* VE

third interspace leads: Arabic numeral followed by capital *V* with subscript arabic numeral. If subscripting is not available, enter the numeral in the same point size on-line with the *V*, with no space between.

$3V_1$, $3V_2$, $3V_3$, etc.
or 3V1, 3V2, 3V3, etc.

esophageal leads: Capital *E* followed by subscript arabic numeral. If subscripting is not available, enter the numeral in the same point size on-line with the *E*, with no space between.

E_{15}, E_{24}, E_{50}, etc.
or E15, E24, E50, etc.

sequential leads: Repeat the *V*, and do not use a hyphen (or dash).

leads V_1 through V_5 *or* V1 through V5
not V_1 through $_5$ *or* V1 through 5
not V_1-V_5 *or* V1-V5
not V_{1-5} *or* V1-5

tracing terms
In general, for electrocardiographic deflections, use all capitals, but larger and smaller Q, R, and S waves may be differentiated by capital and lowercased letters, respectively. Do not place a hyphen after the single letter except when the term is used as an adjective.

Q wave, q wave
QS wave, qs wave
R wave, r wave
S wave, s wave
R' wave, r' wave
S' wave, s' wave
Q-wave pathology

Some additional tracing terms follow. For terms such as *P wave*, in which there is no hyphen, insert a hyphen when the term is used as an adjective (*P-wave pathology*).

J junction
J point
P wave
QT interval, prolongation, etc.

QT$_c$ (if subscript not available, express as *QTc* or *corrected
   QT interval*)
PR interval, segment, etc.
QRS axis, complex, configuration, etc.
ST segment, depression, etc.
ST-T segment, elevation, etc.
T wave
Ta wave
U wave

Note: For *QRS axis,* use a plus or a minus sign followed by arabic
numerals and a degree sign to express the number of degrees, e.g.,
QRS +60°. If the degree sign is not available, write out *degrees:*
QRS +60 degrees.

heart sounds and murmurs
   Abbreviate heart sounds and components as follows, using subscript
numerals if available; otherwise, place numerals on-line.

first heart sound	S_1 *or* S1
second heart sound	S_2 *or* S2
third heart sound	S_3 *or* S3
fourth heart sound	S_4 *or* S4
aortic valve component	A_2 *or* A2
mitral valve component	M_1 *or* M1
pulmonic valve component	P_2 *or* P2
tricuspid valve component	T_1 *or* T1

Express murmurs with arabic numerals 1 to 4 for diastolic murmurs,
1 to 6 for systolic murmurs, (from soft or low grade to loud or high grade).
Roman numerals are not acceptable.

grade 1	barely audible, must strain to hear
grade 2	quiet, but clearly audible
grade 3	moderately loud
grade 4	loud
grade 5	very loud; audible with stethoscope partly off the chest
grade 6	so loud that it can be heard with stethoscope just above chest wall

Place a virgule between the diastolic and systolic grades. Express
partial units as indicated.

grade 1/4 murmur

D: grade 4 and a half over 6 murmur
T: grade 4.5 over 6 murmur

D: grade 4 to 5 over 6 murmur
T: grade 4 to 5 over 6 murmur
or grade 4/6 to 5/6 murmur

Extend murmur names and descriptions even when they are abbreviated in dictation.

ASM	atrial systolic murmur
CM	continuous murmur
DM	diastolic murmur
DSM	delayed systolic murmur
ESM	ejection systolic murmur
IDM	immediate diastolic murmur
LSM	late systolic murmur
PSM	pansystolic murmur
SDM	systolic-diastolic murmur
SEM	systolic ejection murmur
SM	systolic murmur

D: to-and-fro SDM
T: to-and-fro systolic-diastolic murmur

A bruit is an abnormal sound or murmur heard on auscultation. The plural form is *bruits*.
Spell out the following abbreviations even when they are dictated in phonocardiographic tracings.

AEC	aortic ejection click
AOC	aortic opening click
C	click
E	ejection sound
EC	ejection click
NEC	nonejection click
PEC	pulmonary ejection click
OS	opening snap
SC	systolic click
SS	summation sound
W	whoop

NYHA classification of cardiac failure
Widely adopted classification of cardiac failure that was developed
by **N**ew **Y**ork **H**eart **A**ssociation. Lowercase *class*; use roman numerals
I through *IV.*

I   asymptomatic
II   comfortable at rest, symptomatic with normal activity
III   comfortable at rest, symptomatic with less than normal activity
IV   severe cardiac failure, symptomatic at rest

DIAGNOSIS
Cardiac failure, class III.

pacemaker codes
Capitalize these three-letter codes, without spaces or periods.

AVD

First and second letters refer to:

A   atrium
V   ventricle
D   both atrium and ventricle
O   neither atrium nor ventricle

Third letter refers to:

I   inhibited response
T   triggered response
D   inhibited and triggered response
O   no response

categories
See
cancer classifications
classifications
names
scales
scores

Catterall hip score
　　See scores

Caucasian
　　Always capitalize.

　　This is a 59-year-old Caucasian female.

　　See sociocultural designations

cavities, body
　　See body cavities

cc
　　Abbreviation for *cubic centimeter,* for *carbon copy*, and for *courtesy copy*. No periods are used for any of these meanings.

　　See copy designation

cedilla accent mark (ç)
　　See accent marks

Celsius (C)
　　See
　　International System of Measuring Units
　　temperature, temperature scales

Centers for Disease Control
　　A consortium of US Public Health Service agencies whose purpose is to control infectious and other preventable diseases. Note plural: *Centers* not *Center.* Abbreviation: CDC (no periods).

centi-
 Inseparable prefix denoting one hundred, or one-hundredth of a unit. To convert to basic unit, move decimal point two places to the left.

 256 centimeters = 2.56 meters

centigrade
 See temperature, temperature scales

centigray (cGy)
 One-hundredth of a gray, the SI (International System of Measuring Units) unit of absorbed dose of ionizing radiation. Abbreviation: cGy (no periods).

centimeter (cm)
 One-hundredth of a meter. Also equal to 10 millimeters. To convert to inches, multiply by 0.4. Abbreviation: cm (no period).

 160 cm = 64 inches

cents
 See money

centuries
 See years, decades, centuries

Certification Commission
 See Medical Transcriptionist Certification Program at AAMT

certification designations
 See credentials, professional

certification examination
 See Medical Transcriptionist Certification Program at AAMT

certified medical transcriptionist (CMT)

Professional designation awarded after meeting certification requirements as specified by Medical Transcriptionist Certification Program at
AAMT. Abbreviation: CMT (no periods).

See
CMT
credentials, professional
Medical Transcriptionist Certification Program at AAMT

cervical intraepithelial neoplasia

Abbreviation: CIN (no periods).

See cancer classifications

cesarean section

See obstetrics terminology

chair, chairperson

Preferred to *chairman* or *chairwoman*.

See sexist language

character

Any letter, number, symbol, or function key necessary for the final
appearance and content of a document, including the space bar, carriage
return, underscore, bold, and any character contained within a macro,
header, or footer. AAMT prefers the character as the basic unit of
measure, where such measures are appropriate.

See
Appendix F, "AAMT Explores Quality and Quantity Issues"
character spacing
line counts

character spacing

Use a single character space **following**

- each word (unless the next character is a punctuation mark, in which case the space follows the punctuation mark)

- a comma

- a semicolon

- a period at the end of a sentence

- a period at the end of an abbreviation

- a question mark

- an exclamation mark

- a colon used as a punctuation mark

- a closing quotation mark

- a closing parenthesis (unless the next character is a punctuation mark, in which case the space follows the punctuation mark)

- a closing bracket (unless the next character is a punctuation mark, in which case the space follows the punctuation mark)

Note: The traditional use of two spaces at the end of a sentence, i.e., after a period, question mark, or exclamation mark, and after a colon, continues to be acceptable. However, the use of computers and word processors has led to such widespread use of the single space instead that single-spacing is becoming more common, even preferred.

If you have not already made the transition to single-spacing, you may be resistant to doing so. You may find it awkward at first, but if you persist, it will become routine both in the doing and in the viewing. And consider this: Typeset materials (newspapers, books, magazines) routinely use single-spacing, and we accept it without notice or comment.

Use a single character space **between**

- words or symbols

- a word or symbol and an opening quotation mark

- a word or symbol and an opening parenthesis

- a word or symbol and an opening bracket

> *If it were not for space, all matter would*
> *be jammed together in one lump and*
> *that lump wouldn't take up any room.*
> Irene Peter

Do not use a character space **before or after**

- an apostrophe (except when the apostrophe ends the term, as in a plural possessive, e.g., *patients'*, in which case a space follows the apostrophe unless it is followed by another punctuation mark)

- a colon used in expressions of time, e.g., 12:45

- a colon used in expressions of equator positions, e.g., 1:30

- a colon used in expressions of ratios, e.g. 1:4

- a colon used in expressions of dilutions, e.g., 1:100,000

- a comma in numeric expressions, e.g., 12,034

- a decimal point in numeric expressions (except in those rare instances when a unit less than 1 does not call for a zero to be placed before the decimal, e.g., .22-caliber rifle, in which instances a space precedes the decimal point but does not follow it)

- a decimal point in expressions of dollars and cents, e.g., $1.50

- a hyphen, e.g., 3-0

- a dash

- a virgule, e.g., 2/6

- a period within an abbreviation, e.g., q.i.d.

- an ampersand in abbreviations such as T&A, D&C

  Do not use a character space **after**

- an opening quotation mark

- an opening parenthesis

- a word followed by a punctuation mark

- a decimal point in numeric expressions

  Do not use a character space **before**

- a punctuation mark (except an opening parenthesis, bracket, brace, or quotation mark)

  See character

chemical nomenclature

chemical names
Do not capitalize chemical names.

acetylsalicylic acid

concentration
Use brackets to express chemical concentration. When concentrations are expressed as percentages, use the percent sign rather than the spelled-out form; do not use brackets.

$[HCO_3^-]$
15% HNO_3

elements and compounds
Do not capitalize the names of chemical elements and compounds written in full. Always use the name rather than the symbol at the

beginning of a sentence. Never use a hyphen in chemical elements or compounds, whether used as nouns or adjectives.

carbon dioxide
potassium
carbon monoxide poisoning

formulas
Use parentheses for innermost units, adding brackets, then braces, if necessary. Italics may also be used for some portions. Consult appropriate references.

The chemical formula for chlorphenoxamine hydrochloride:
2-[1-(4-chlorophenyl)-1-phenylethoxy]-*N,N*-dimethylethanamine hydrochloride

The chemical formula for hydroxychloroquine sulfate:
7-chloro-4-{4-[ethyl(2-hydroxyethyl)amino]-1-methylbutylamino}-quinoline sulfate

symbols
Use chemical symbols when the terms are accompanied by quantities or in reference to laboratory data. Capitalize the initial letter of the symbol of each chemical element. Replace subscripted and superscripted numerals with on-line regular-sized numerals when word processing equipment does not allow accurate subscripting and superscripting. Never use periods or other punctuation with chemical symbols.

oxygen, O_2
carbon dioxide, CO_2
NaCl
Na_2SO_4

biochemical terminology
Since abbreviations for biochemical terminology may not be readily recognized by healthcare professionals, write out such terms in patient records. Use their abbreviated forms only in tables and in communications among biochemical specialists.

*examples of biochemical groups, terms, and abbreviations
(3-letter and / or 1-letter)*

amino acids of proteins	phenylalanine	Phe, F
	proline	Pro, P
	tryptophan	Trp, W
bases and nucleosides	cytosine	Cyt
	purine	Pur
	uracil	Ura
common ribonucleosides	adenosine	Ado, A
	cytidine	Cyd, C
	uridine	Urd, U
sugars and carbohydrates	fructose	Fru
	glucose	Rib

See
abbreviations
drug terminology
pH
subscripts
superscripts

Chicano

Usage and acceptance of this designation for a Mexican-American is preferred by some, considered derogatory by others. Plural form: *Chicanos*. Widely preferred alternative is *Mexican-American*.

See
Mexican-American
sociocultural designations

chief, Chief

Capitalize only if it is a formal title and it precedes a name; otherwise, lowercase.

Chief Watson
The chief called an emergency meeting.

See titles

child, children
    See age referents

Child classification of hepatic risk criteria
    See classifications

chromosomal terms
    See genetics terminology

church, Church
    Capitalize only when used in the proper name of an organization, building, congregation, or denomination; otherwise, lowercase.

    St. Mary's Church
    the Cornerstone Baptist Church
    a Methodist church
    the church
    Church of England
    Church of Jesus Christ of Latter-day Saints (*note that* day *is lowercased*)

CIN grades
    See cancer classifications

circumflex accent mark (^)
    See accent marks

city
    See
    Appendix CC, "State Names and Abbreviations, Major Cities, and State/City Resident Designations"
    state, county, city, and town names and resident designations
    USPS guidelines

Clark level
    See cancer classifications

class

> *See*
> cancer classifications
> classifications

classifications

Systematic arrangements into groups or classes. Check appropriate references for guidance not provided below.

burn classifications

Burns are described as first, second, third, and fourth degree, according to the depth of burn. A hyphen in the adjective form is acceptable (e.g., first-degree burn) but not required, so AAMT recommends dropping it. Ordinals are acceptable; do not use hyphens: 1st, 2nd, 3rd, and 4th degree burns.

Rule of Nines: Formula, based on multiples of 9, for determining percentage of burned body surface. (Does not apply to children because the head is disproportionately large.)

head	9%
each arm	9%
each leg	18%
anterior trunk	18%
posterior trunk	18%
perineum	1%

Berkow formula: Rule of Nines adjusted for patient's age. Assigns a higher percentage to a child's head, which is larger than an adult's head.

Child classification of hepatic risk criteria

Classification of operative risk. Capitalize *Child* (eponymic term), lowercase *class,* capitalize the letter that follows.

> Child class A
> Child class B
> Child class C

diabetes mellitus classifications

> *See* diabetes mellitus terminology

fracture classifications
LeFort fractures: Classification of facial fractures. Use roman numerals I, II, or III. Do not space between *Le* and *Fort*.

LeFort I
LeFort II
LeFort III

Salter fractures: Classification of epiphyseal fractures. Express by roman numerals I (least severe) through VI (most severe).

Salter III

Check appropriate references for additional fracture classification systems.

Hunt and Hess neurological classification
Classifies prognosis of patients with hemorrhage. Write out and lowercase *grade;* do not abbreviate. Use arabic numerals 1 through 4.

grade 1
grade 2
grade 3
grade 4

NYHA classification of cardiac failure
See cardiology terminology

physical status classification
A classification developed by the American Society of Anesthesiologists to classify risk of complications for patients undergoing surgery. Lowercase *class* and use arabic numerals (1 through 5); add the capital letter E to indicate an emergency operation.

class 1E

See
cancer classifications
names
scales
scores

clauses

A clause is a group of words with a subject and verb and that is a part of a sentence.

independent clause

Also known as *main clause* or *principal clause*. It can stand alone as a sentence. Use a comma to separate independent clauses joined by a conjunction (*and, but, for, or, nor, yet,* or *so*). The comma is optional if the main clauses are short and their meanings will not be confused. Use a semicolon instead of a comma when the second clause is closely linked to the first without a conjunction, or when one or both of the independent clauses have internal commas. A colon may be used instead of a semicolon to separate two independent clauses when the second one explains or expands upon the first. *See* dependent clause *below.*

> The patient came into the emergency room.
> The platysma was then divided in the direction of its fibers, and blunt dissection was performed so that the prevertebral space was entered.
> A consultation was obtained, and liver function studies were done.

> He had numerous complaints; several were inconsistent with one another.
> *or* He had numerous complaints: several were inconsistent with one another.

dependent clause

One that is subordinate to or depends on the independent clause; also known as a subordinate clause. It has a subject and a verb, but it cannot stand alone; hence, its name. It may be introduced by such terms as *who, whom, that, which, when, after, although, before, if, whether. See* independent clause *above.*

In the following example, the dependent clause is in italics.

> The gallbladder, *although it was inflamed,* was without stones.

dependent essential clause

Dependent clause that cannot be eliminated without changing the meaning of the sentence; also known as restrictive clause. Use *who* or *whom* to introduce an essential clause referring to a human being or to an animal with a name. Use *that* or *which* to introduce an essential clause referring to an inanimate object or to an animal without a name.

Exception: When *that* as a conjunction is used elsewhere in the same sentence, use *which,* not *that,* to introduce an essential clause. Do not use commas to set off dependent essential clauses. *See* dependent nonessential clause *below.*

In the following sentences, the essential clauses are in italics.

The patient came into the emergency room, and she was treated for tachycardia *that had resisted conversion in her physician's office.* She had two large wounds *that were bleeding profusely* and several small bleeders.

dependent nonessential clause
Dependent clause that can be eliminated without changing the meaning of the sentence; also known as nonrestrictive clause. Use commas to set off nonessential subordinate clauses or nonessential participial phrases. Use *who* or *whom* to introduce a nonessential clause referring to a human being or an animal with a name. Use *which* to introduce a nonessential clause referring to an inanimate object or to an animal without a name. *See* dependent essential clause *above.*

The patient, *who was referred by her family physician,* came into the emergency room.
The patient's parents, *who had been summoned from Europe,* were consulted about his past history.
The incision, *which ran from the umbilicus to the symphysis pubis,* was closed in layers.
The operation, *which began at 7 a.m.,* took 17 hours.

coordinate clause
One that is the same type as another (main to main, dependent to dependent). The following sentence has two main coordinate clauses separated by a comma and *and.*

The patient came into the emergency room, and she was treated for tachycardia.

main clause
See independent clause *above.*

nonrestrictive clause
See dependent nonessential clause *above.*

principal clause
　　See independent clause *above.*

restrictive clause
　　See dependent essential clause *above.*

subordinate clause
　　See dependent clause *above.*

　　See
　　conjunctions
　　phrases
　　sentences

cliches
　　See jargon

*At the beginning there was the Word—
at the end just the Cliché.*
Stanislaw J. Lec

clipped sentences
　　See sentences

clock referents
　　Sometimes an anatomic position is described in terms of clockface orientation as seen by the viewer. Use *o'clock* in such instances.

　　The incision was made at the 3 o'clock position.

clotting factor terms
　　Lowercase *factor* and use roman numerals.

factor I	fibrinogen
factor II	prothrombin
factor III	thromboplastin
factor IV	calcium ions
factor V	proaccelerin
factor VI	(none currently designated)
factor VII	proconvertin
factor VIII	antihemophilic factor
factor IX	Christmas factor
factor X	Stuart factor
factor XI	plasma thromboplastin antecedent
factor XII	glass factor
factor XIII	fibrin-stabilizing factor

Add a lowercased *a* to designate a factor's activated form.

factor Xa

New terms for factor XIII and von Willebrand factor are preferred, but older terms continue to be used. Transcribe the dictated form, expressing it appropriately.

old	*new*
factor VIII:C	factor VIII
factor VIII:CAg	factor VIII:Ag
von Willebrand factor	vWF
factor VIII:RAg	vWF:Ag
VIII:RCoF	riatocetin cofactor

Use arabic numerals for platelet factors (abbreviation: PF).

platelet factor 3	PF 3

CMT

Abbreviation for the professional credential *certified medical transcriptionist*. The term and its abbreviation apply only to those who have met the requirements of the Medical Transcriptionist Certification Program at AAMT.

Use capital letters for the abbreviation. Do not use periods. Lowercase the extended form.

CMT *but* certified medical transcriptionist

Do not link *CMT* to another professional or academic designation by a virgule or hyphen; rather, place a comma and space between them.

Sharon Rhodes, CMT, ART *not* Sharon Rhodes CMT/ART

Do not use *CMT* after the personal initials for a transcriptionist. (Likewise, do not add MD to a dictator's initials.)

db:jb *not* db:jbcmt *not* dbmd:jbcmt

The abbreviations *MT* (medical transcriptionist) and *MLS* (medical language specialist) should be used only in a generic sense. It is inappropriate to use either abbreviation after one's name because doing so gives the impression it carries the weight of a professional certification designation. CMT is the only recognized professional certification designation for medical transcriptionists, and it may be used only if authorized through the Medical Transcriptionist Certification Program at AAMT.

Note: Other certifications are also designated by the abbreviation CMT, e.g., certified massage therapist, certified music therapist.

See
credentials, professional
degrees, academic
MLS
MT
Medical Transcriptionist Certification Program at AAMT

Co.
See business names

coagulation factors
See clotting factor terms

coast, Coast
See north, south, east, west

code, coding

code
A number or a number-letter combination assigned to a diagnosis or procedure or other terminology. Used for reimbursement, research, and statistical purposes. Coding systems include ICD-9-CM, SNOMED, DSM-III-R.

0.74.21   Coxsackie pericarditis

coding
Process of assigning codes for reimbursement, research, or statistical purposes.

coined terms
Terms made up by the dictator. Avoid as much as possible. Many are back-formations.

See
back-formations
editing
jargon

collective nouns
See nouns

college, College
Capitalize only when part of a proper name.

Modesto Junior College
Delta College
community college
college bookstore
college student

colons (:)
The primary function of a colon as a punctuation mark is to introduce what follows: a list, series, or enumeration; an example; sometimes a quotation (instead of a comma).

She said: "I have never gotten along with my mother, and I no longer try."
or She said, "I have never gotten along with my mother, and I no longer try."

Do not use a colon to introduce words that fit properly into the grammatical structure of the sentence without the colon, for example, after a verb, between a preposition and its object, or after *because*.

The patient is using Theo-Dur, prednisone, and Bronkometer.
The patient is *on* Theo-Dur, prednisone, and Bronkometer.
He came to the emergency room *because* he was experiencing fever and chills of several hours' duration.

Capitalize the word following the colon if it is normally capitalized, if it follows a heading or subheading, or if the list or series that follows the colon includes multiple complete sentences or thoughts separated by periods. Lowercase the first letter of each item in a series following a colon when the items are separated by commas.

The patient is on the following medications: Theo-Dur, prednisone, Bronkometer.
ABDOMEN: Benign.
Pelvic examination revealed the following: Moderately atrophic vulva. Markedly atrophic vaginal mucosa.
or Pelvic examination revealed the following: moderately atrophic vulva, markedly atrophic vaginal mucosa.

A colon may be used instead of a semicolon to separate two main clauses when the second one explains or expands upon the first.

He had numerous complaints; several were inconsistent with one another.
or He had numerous complaints: several were inconsistent with one another.

The colon is also used in equator readings, ratios, and time expressions. It may introduce a series or follow a heading or subheading, and it may replace a dash in some instances.

See
dashes
equator readings

formats
ratio
series
time

coma scale, Glasgow
See scales

commas

Commas are used to indicate a break in thought, to set off material, and to introduce a new but connected thought.

Sometimes commas **must** be used; sometimes they **must not** be used; sometimes their use is **optional**. The trend is toward avoiding overuse. Use commas when the rules require them and when they enhance clarity, improve readability, or diminish confusion or misunderstanding.

See specific entries, including
addresses
adjectives
appositives
clauses
conjunctions
credentials, professional
dates
degrees, academic
elliptical construction
International System of Measuring Units
laboratory data and values
Latin abbreviations
numbers
parentheses
parenthetical expressions
phrases
quotations, quotation marks
sentences
series
state, county, city, and town names and resident designations
titles
units of measure

company names

In military uses, capitalize *company* only when it is part of a name; do not abbreviate it.

Company C *not* Co. C

See business names

compass directions

See
addresses
north, south, east, west

complement factors

Factors involved in antigen-antibody reactions and inflammations. Immediately follow a capital *C, B, P,* or *D* with an on-line arabic number.

C1
C7

For fragments of complement components, add a lowercased letter (usually *a* or *b*).

C5a
Bb

compound modifiers

A compound modifier is two or more words that act as a unit modifying a noun or pronoun. The use of hyphens varies depending on the type of compound modifier, as indicated below.

Some compound modifiers are so commonly used together that they are automatically read as a unit and do not need to be joined with hyphens.

deep tendon reflexes
jugular venous distention
left lower quadrant
low back pain

Do not use hyphens in compound modifiers that are clear without them.

dark brown lesion

adjective ending in ly
Do use a hyphen in a compound modifier beginning with an adjective ending in *ly*. (This requires distinguishing between adjectives ending in *ly* and adverbs ending in *ly;* compound modifiers containing an adverb ending in *ly* do not take a hyphen.)

scholarly-looking patient
squirrelly-faced stuffed animal
but quickly paced steps

adjective-noun compound
Use a hyphen in an adjective-noun compound that precedes and modifies another noun. *See* noun-adjective compound *below.*

second-floor office
but The office is on the second floor.

adjective with preposition
Use hyphens in most compound adjectives that contain a preposition.

figure-of-eight
finger-to-nose

adjective with participle
Use a hyphen to join an adjective to a participle, whether the compound precedes or follows the noun.

good-natured, soft-spoken patient
The patient is good-natured and soft-spoken.

adverb with participle or adjective
Use a hyphen to form a compound modifier made up of an adverb coupled with a participle or adjective when they precede the noun they modify but not when they follow it.

well-developed and well-nourished male
but The patient was well developed and well nourished.

fast-acting medication
but The medication is fast acting.

adverb ending in ly
Do not use a hyphen in a compound modifier to link an adverb ending in *ly* with a participle or adjective.

recently completed workup
moderately acute pain
financially stable investment

adverb preceding a compound modifier
Do not use a hyphen in a compound modifier preceded by an adverb.

somewhat well nourished patient

adverb with very
Drop the hyphen in a compound modifier with a participle or adjective when it is preceded by the adverb *very.*

very well developed patient

disease-entity modifiers
Do not use hyphens with most disease-entity modifiers even when they precede the noun. Check appropriate references for guidance.

cervical disk disease
oat cell carcinoma
pelvic inflammatory disease
sickle cell disease
urinary tract infection
but insulin-dependent diabetes mellitus *and* non-insulin-dependent diabetes mellitus

eponyms
Use a hyphen to join two or more eponymic names used as multiple-word modifiers of operations, procedures, instruments, etc. Do not use a hyphen if the eponymic name refers to a single person. Use appropriate references to differentiate.

Osgood-Schlatter disease
Chevalier Jackson forceps

equal, complementary, or contrasting adjectives
Use a hyphen to join two adjectives that are equal, complementary, or contrasting when they precede or follow the noun they modify.

anterior-posterior infarction
physician-patient confidentiality issues
His eyes are blue-green.

foreign expressions
Do not hyphenate foreign expressions used in compound adjectives, even when they precede the noun they modify (unless they are always hyphenated).

in vitro experiments
carcinoma in situ
cul-de-sac *(always hyphenated)*
ex officio member

high- and low-
Use a hyphen in most *high-* and *low-* compound adjectives.

high-density mass
low-frequency waves

noun-adjective compound
Sometimes a hyphen joins a noun-adjective compound but not always. Usage governs, so check appropriate references. When a hyphen is used, it is used whether the noun-adjective compound precedes or follows the noun it is modifying.

It is a medication-resistant condition.
or The condition was medication-resistant.

This is a symptom-free patient.
or The patient was symptom-free.

noun with participle
Use a hyphen to join a noun and a participle to form a compound modifier preceding a noun.

bone-biting forceps
pus-aspirating methods
mucus-coated throat *(the throat was coated with* mucus, *not* mucous)
callus-forming lesion *(the lesion was forming* callus, *not* callous)

numerals with words
Use a hyphen when numbers are used with words as a compound modifier preceding a noun.

5-cm incision
3-week history

proper nouns as adjective
Do not use hyphens in proper nouns even when they serve as a modifier preceding a noun.

South American countries
John F. Kennedy High School

Do not use hyphens in combinations of proper noun and common noun serving as a modifier.

Tylenol capsule administration

series of hyphenated compound modifiers
Use a suspensive hyphen after each incomplete modifier when there is a series of hyphenated compound modifiers with a common last word that is expressed only after the final modifier in the series. If one or more of the incomplete modifiers is not hyphenated, repeat the base with each, hyphenating or not, as appropriate.

10- to 12-year history
full- and split-thickness grafts
preoperative and postoperative diagnoses (*not* pre- and
    postoperative diagnoses)

to clarify or to avoid confusion
Use a hyphen to clarify meaning and to avoid confusion, absurdity, or ambiguity in compound modifiers.

large-bowel obstruction (*obstruction of the large bowel,* not *a large obstruction of the bowel*)

compound modifiers formed from compound modifiers
Use a hyphen or en dash to join hyphenated compound modifiers or a hyphenated compound modifier with a one-word modifier.

non-insulin-dependent diabetes (*from* insulin-dependent diabetes)
or non–insulin-dependent diabetes

Use a hyphen or en dash to join two unhyphenated compound modifiers.

the North Carolina-South Carolina border
or the North Carolina–South Carolina border

Use a hyphen or en dash to join an unhyphenated and a hyphenated compound modifier.

The patient is French Canadian-African-American.
or The patient is French Canadian–African-American.

Use a hyphen or en dash to join an unhyphenated compound modifier with a one-word modifier.

vitamin D-deficiency rickets
or vitamin D–deficiency rickets

diabetes mellitus-related symptoms
or diabetes mellitus–related symptoms

credit card-operated kiosk
or credit card–operated kiosk

See
adjectives
adverbs
compound words
dashes
hyphens
letters
numbers
prefixes

compound words
Compound words may be written as one or multiple words; check appropriate references.

hyphens

Hyphens are always used in some compound words, sometimes in others, never in others. Check appropriate references for guidance.

> father-in-law
> cul-de-sac
> vice president
> president-elect
> chief of staff
> attorney at law
> ex officio

Use a hyphen to join two nouns that are equal, complementary, or contrasting.

> blood-brain barrier
> secretary-treasurer
> fracture-dislocation

Do not hyphenate proper nouns of more than one word, even when they serve as a modifier preceding a noun.

> South American countries
> John F. Kennedy High School

Do not use a hyphen in a combination of proper noun and common noun.

> Tylenol capsule administration

Use a hyphen with all compound nouns containing *ex-* when *ex-* means former and precedes a noun that can stand on its own.

> ex-president
> ex-student

Use a hyphen in compound verbs unless one of the terms is a preposition.

> single-space
> *but* follow up

Sometimes hyphenated compound words become so well established that the hyphen is dropped and the words are joined together without a hyphen. When such a word can be used as either a noun, adjective, or verb, the noun and adjective forms are joined without a hyphen, but the verb form remains two separate words if one of them is a preposition.

noun, adjective	*verb*
checkup	check up
followup	follow up
workup	work up
followthrough	follow through

The patient was lost to followup.
I will follow up the patient in three weeks.

plurals

For those written as a single word, form the plural by adding *s*.

fingerbreadths
tablespoonfuls
workups

For those formed by a noun and modifier(s), form the plural by making the noun plural.

sisters-in-law

For compound nouns containing a possessive, make the second noun plural.

associate's degrees
The driver's licenses were ...

For some compound nouns, the plural is formed irregularly.

touch-me-nots

Some terms consisting of a word followed by a single letter or symbol are hyphenated; others are not. Check appropriate references for guidance.

type I
vitamin D
LeFort I
Dukes A

Some terms with a single letter or symbol followed by a word are hyphenated, others are not. Some terms may be unhyphenated in their noun form but hyphenated in their adjective form. Check appropriate references for guidance.

B-complex vitamins
T cell
T-cell abnormality
T wave
T-wave abnormality
x-rays
x-ray results

When a Greek letter is part of the name, use a hyphen after the symbol but not after the spelled-out form.

ß-carotene *but* beta carotene

possessive forms
Use 's after the last word in a hyphenated compound term.

daughter-in-law's inquiry

See
compound modifiers
dashes
hyphens
letters
numbers
prefixes

confidentiality

Each patient has a legal and ethical right to confidentiality. Confidentiality is a quality of private information that is developed by or derived from the patient with the explicit promise or the reasonable expectation that it will not be disclosed except for the purposes (such as receiving healthcare services) for which it was provided.

Confidentiality is sometimes confused with two related but different concepts: privacy and privilege. *Privacy* means an individual's right to be left alone and/or to decide what to share with others. Privacy may, for example, affect whether gratuitous, irrelevant, and personal information is even included in a record. *Privilege* means the legal protection against being forced to violate confidentiality in a legal proceeding, such as by disclosing confidential records.

Medical transcriptionists share with other healthcare personnel the responsibility to respect the confidentiality of medical records. Principally state laws, but also federal laws, can govern the extent of confidentiality. There are many exceptions, under which disclosure can be legally required.

There are an increasing number of lawsuits over violations of confidentiality. Care in preserving the routine confidentiality of records is an important element of risk management.

See
Appendix G, "Can You Keep a Secret?"
Appendix H, "Healthcare Reform and Confidentiality"
release of information
risk management

congestive heart failure classification
See cardiology terminology

conjunctions
Words such as *and, but, for, or, nor, yet, so* that join words, phrases, or clauses, thereby indicating their relationship.

conjunctive adverbs
Connect two independent clauses. They include *consequently, finally, furthermore, however, moreover, nevertheless, similarly, subsequently, then, therefore, thus.* Precede a conjunctive adverb by a semicolon (sometimes a period), and follow it by a comma.

He was admitted through the emergency room; consequently, he was taken to surgery.
She reported feeling better; however, her fever still spiked in the evenings.

coordinating conjunctions (and, but, or, nor, for)
Join separate main clauses. They are usually preceded by a comma, sometimes by a semicolon, occasionally a colon.

He was seen in the emergency room, but he was not admitted.

Do not use a comma before a coordinating conjunction that is followed by a second verb without a new subject.

> The patient tolerated the procedure well and left the department in stable condition.
> The gallbladder was inflamed but without stones.

subordinate conjunctions (while, where, since, after, yet, so)
Precede by a comma.

> He was in great pain, yet he refused treatment.

correlative conjunctions
Terms or phrases used in pairs, e.g., *either...or, neither...nor,* and *not only...but also.*

> *See*
> clauses
> either...or, neither...nor
> not only...but also
> phrases
> sentences
> that

consensus
Note spelling. The term, derived from *consent* (not *census*), means an agreement or decision reached by a group as a whole (they consent).
The phrase *consensus of opinion* is redundant; *consensus* is adequate.

consonants
Letters other than vowels; therefore, all letters except *a, e, i, o, u* (and sometimes *y*).

consultation report
A consultation includes examination, review, and assessment of a patient by a healthcare provider other than the attending physician. The report generated is called a consultation report, which is one of the basic 4 reports. The consulting specialist directs the report to the physician requesting the consultation, usually the attending physician.

Content usually includes patient examination, review, and assessment. It may be prepared in letter or report format.

> *See*
> Appendix A, "Sample Reports"
> basic 4 reports
> formats

continual, continuous

Do not confuse the terms. *Continual* means recurring frequently; *continuous* means going on without interruption.

> She sneezed continually.
> He was on continuous-flow oxygen.

continuation pages

See formats

contractions

Words with missing letters or numbers denoted by apostrophes. They make a professional document look casual, so avoid them except in direct quotations.

dictated	*transcribed*
can't	cannot
I'd	I would
he's	he is
it's	it is

Extend abbreviations that contain contractions.

> D: The patient OD'd on ...
> T: The patient overdosed on ...

When you use contractions, take care to place the apostrophe accurately.

> The mother reported, "He's been hysterical."

Apostrophes are omitted in contractions that have become such commonly used brief forms that they are themselves considered full terms.

plane (*from* airplane)
phone (*from* telephone)

See apostrophes

copy designation
Notation of those to whom copies of a report or letter are to be distributed. Place copy designations flush left and two line spaces below the end of the report.

bc	blind copy
cc	carbon copy, courtesy copy
c	copy
pc	photocopy

A blind copy designation is noted only on the file copy and on the copy to whom it is sent; other recipients' copies do not indicate the blind copy (thus, its name).

Corp.
See business names

county names
See state, county, city, and town names and resident designations

courtesy copy
See copy designation

courtesy titles
See titles

cranial nerves

Roman numerals remain preferred, but arabic numerals are increasingly acceptable for cranial nerve designations. Be consistent. (Physician, employer, or client will often indicate preference.)

cranial nerve XII   cranial nerve 12
cranial nerves II-XII   cranial nerves 2-12

Ordinals may be written out or expressed in numeric form (arabic, of course).

fourth cranial nerve
or 4th cranial nerve

English and Latin names

English names are preferred to Latin, but transcribe Latin forms if they are dictated.

number	English name	Latin name
I *or* 1	olfactory	olfactorius
II *or* 2	optic	opticus
III *or* 3	oculomotor	oculomotorius
IV *or* 4	trochlear	trochlearis
V *or* 5	trigeminal	trigeminus
VI *or* 6	abducens	abducens
VII *or* 7	facial	facialis
VIII *or* 8	acoustic	vestibulocochlearis
IX *or* 9	glossopharyngeal	glossopharyngeus
X *or* 10	vagus	vagus
XI *or* 11	accessory	accessorius
XII *or* 12	hypoglossal	hypoglossus

credentials, professional

Designations, such as *MD, CMT, RRA,* that identify the professional degrees, certifications, licensures, or registrations carried by the individual.

abbreviated forms

Use abbreviated forms after a full name (not just a surname). Do not use periods in most such abbreviations; follow the preferred style for the designation. Use commas to set off professional credentials when they follow the person's name.

William Walters, MD
Stella Olson, CMT, AAMT director

capitalization
Capitalize abbreviated forms, but do not capitalize extended forms.

Jana Tesch, CMT *but* Jana Tesch, a certified medical transcriptionist

with initials
Do not use credentials after initials, as in dictator-transcriptionist initials at the end of a report.

JD:DH *not* JDMD:DHCMT

false credentials
Occasionally, individuals will follow their name by an abbreviation that is not a recognized professional credential. Doing so gives the appearance of presenting the abbreviation as a recognized professional credential. Whether or not such usage is intended to deceive, it should be avoided.

Mary Frank
not Mary Frank, MT
not Mary Frank, MLS

multiple credentials
If the individual holds multiple professional credentials, present them in the order preferred by the individual, with a comma (not a virgule) and a space between them.

Marilyn Craddock, CMT, RRA *not* Marilyn Craddock, CMT/RRA

salutations
Do not use credentials in salutations.

Dear Ms. Heath: *not* Dear Ms. Heath, CMT:

See
CMT
degrees, academic

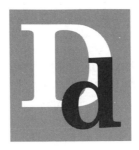

D

    D as abbreviation for *dictated* is used throughout this text to indicate what was dictated and to contrast it with what should be transcribed (*T*).

dangling modifiers

    A dangling modifier is one whose placement links it to the wrong term or leaves it "dangling" without a reference point. Also known as a *displaced modifier* or *unattached modifier,* it can take any form, e.g., adjective, infinitive, clause, appositive. Dangling participles are most common.

> Entering the abdomen through a Pfannenstiel incision, the omentum was noted to be bound down by adhesions.

    It could be argued that dangling modifiers (particularly dangling participles) are so common throughout medical dictation (particularly in surgical reports) that they have become acceptable. Certainly, to edit multiple dangling modifiers in a single report may raise objections from dictators that their style has been tampered with, and it could be unreasonably time consuming. Thus, AAMT reluctantly acknowledges that in many instances it is prudent to transcribe dangling modifiers as dictated, provided they do not confuse or amuse. Nevertheless, we caution transcriptionists to take care to be alert to dangling modifiers and to change the more ludicrous among them.

    Following is the edited version of the example given above.

> The abdomen was entered through a Pfannenstiel incision, and the omentum was noted to be bound down by adhesions.

> *Everything that can be thought of at all can be thought clearly. Anything that can be said can be said clearly.*
> Ludwig Wittgenstein

Some dangling participles have been legitimized because they are so commonly used and familiar; these include *judging, considering, assuming, concerning, given, owing to,* and *provided.*

Provided he follows instructions, he should heal rapidly.
Considering his medical history, his condition is remarkable.

dangling participles

See dangling modifiers

dashes

Dashes have two forms: the em dash (—) and the en dash (–), with the former being longer than the latter and both being longer than the hyphen (-). Each dash has specific uses. Many contemporary keyboards have a specific key (or a combination of keys) for the em dash (—) and for the en dash (–). Nevertheless, dashes are not required in medical transcription, and alternatives are readily available. Even when dashes are acceptable, their use should be minimized, because their overuse creates visual clutter that makes reading difficult.

When dashes are used, do not space before or after them.

abrupt changes in continuity

Use a comma or em dash to introduce an abrupt change in continuity.

The patient agreed to return tomorrow, if he felt like it.
The patient agreed to return tomorrow—if he felt like it.

clauses

Commas are preferred to em dashes to set off clauses that do not have internal commas.

The patient, who had multiple complaints, demanded to be seen immediately.
preferred to The patient—who had multiple complaints—demanded to be seen immediately.

Following are some common uses of the em dash and en dash with alternatives for medical transcription noted.

Use an em dash or double hyphen to represent missing letters or numbers. Be sure to place a space after the em dash or double hyphen representing the ending letters or numbers in a term.

What the h— did he think I would do?

Use a hyphen or en dash following the area code and prefix of a telephone number.

209-551-9317
209–551–9317

Use a hyphen or en dash between the first five and last four digits of a ZIP-plus-four code.

Modesto, CA 95357-6187
Modesto, CA 95357–6317

See
compound modifiers
compound words
formats
hyphens
phrases
series

data, datum

Data is the plural form of *datum,* and it usually takes a plural verb. It should be noted, however, that the use of *data* as a collective noun taking a singular verb is increasing, and it is apt to become more widely accepted. The singular form, *datum,* is seldom used.

The data were collected over a period of several years.
The data demonstrate conclusive evidence that ...
The research data were checked, datum by datum.

date dictated, date transcribed

These dates should be recorded to monitor dictation and transcription patterns as well as to provide legal documentation of when the work (dictation or transcription) was done.

Medical reports are, among other things, legal documents. As part of risk management, dictation and transcription dates should be entered accurately and should not be altered.

Capitalize *D* and *T*, follow each by a colon and appropriate date, using numerals separated by virgules.

D: 4/18/93
T: 4/19/93

See
audit trails
risk management

dates

Write out the name of the month. Express the day of the month and the year with arabic numerals.

She was born March 17, 1994.

punctuation

When the month, day, and year are given in sequence, set off the year by commas. Do not use ordinals.

She was admitted on December 14, 1993, and discharged on January 4, 1994.

Do not use commas when the month and year are given without the day, or when the military date sequence (day, month, year) is used.

She was admitted in December 1993 and discharged in January 1994.
She was admitted on 14 December 1993 and discharged on 4 January 1994.

Do not use punctuation after the year if the date stands alone, as in admission and discharge dates on reports.

Admission date: April 4, 1994
Discharge date: April 5, 1994

ordinals
Use ordinals when the day of the month precedes the month and is preceded by *the;* do not use commas. Do not use ordinals in month/day/year format.

the 4th of April 1994 *not* April 4th, 1994

military style
When the military style is used, the day precedes the month. Use numerals; do not use commas. Write out or abbreviate the month (without periods) and use arabic figures for day and year.

4 April 1994
4 Apr 1994

virgules
In text, do not express dates with numerals separated by virgules or hyphens. Use virgules in dictation and transcription dates.

The patient was previously seen on April 4, 1994.
not The patient was previously seen on 4/4/94.
and not The patient was previously seen on 4-4-94.

D: 4/10/94 *not* 4-10-94
T: 4/12/94 *not* 4-12-94

See
date dictated, date transcribed
days of the week
years, decades, centuries
months
time zones
virgule

daylight time, daylight-saving time
See time zones

days of the week

Capitalize the names of the days of the week. Do not abbreviate them except in tables, where three-letter abbreviations without periods may be used.

Sunday	Sun
Monday	Mon
Tuesday	Tue
Wednesday	Wed
Thursday	Thu
Friday	Fri
Saturday	Sat

When referring to a day in a report, use the day's name and the date. Avoid terms such as *last* Monday or *next* Wednesday. For dates in previous or subsequent years, specify the year.

Omit *on* before the name of a day when this will not cause confusion. Use *on* between a proper name and a day.

His appointment is Wednesday.
preferred to His appointment is on Wednesday.

He saw Dr. White on Tuesday.

See dates

DC

Abbreviation for *Doctor of Chiropractic* degree. Also, two-letter US Postal Service abbreviation for *District of Columbia*.

See
degrees, academic
USPS guidelines

DD

Abbreviation for *Doctor of Divinity* degree.

See degrees, academic

DDS
Abbreviation for *Doctor of Dental Surgery* degree and for *Doctor of Dental Science* degree.

See degrees, academic

de, du, di, d'
See personal names, nicknames, and initials

decades
See
ages
years, decades, centuries

December
See months

deci-
Prefix meaning one-tenth of a unit. To convert to basic unit, move decimal point one place to the left.

18.3 decigrams = 1.83 grams.

decimal point
See decimals, decimal units

decimals, decimal units
Use numerals to express decimal amounts. Use the period as a decimal point or indicator.

metric measurements
Always use the decimal form with metric measurements, even when they are dictated as a fraction.

D: two and a half centimeters
T: 2.5 cm

When whole numbers are dictated, do not add a decimal point and zero; doing so may cause them to be read as larger quantities. This is essential with drug doses because the addition of a decimal point and zero could lead to serious consequences if misread.

2 mg
not 2.0 mg

When the decimal point and zero following a whole number are dictated to emphasize the preciseness of a measurement, e.g., of a pathology specimen or a laboratory value, transcribe them as dictated. Do not, however, insert the decimal point and zero if they are not dictated.

D&T: The specimen measured 4.8 x 2.0 x 3.4 mm.
but
D&T: The specimen measured 4.8 x 2 x 3.4 mm.

For quantities less than 1, place a zero before the decimal point, except when the number could never equal 1 (e.g., in bullet calibers and in certain statistical expressions such as correlation coefficients, statistical probability, etc.).

0.75 mg
.22-caliber rifle

Do not exceed two places following the decimal except in special circumstances, e.g., specific gravity values, or when a precise measurement is intended. *See* nonmetric forms of measure *below.*

specific gravity 1.030

nonmetric forms of measure
Use the decimal form with nonmetric forms of measure when a precise measurement is intended and the fraction form would be both cumbersome and inexact. Three or more places may follow the decimal.

The 0.1816-inch screw was inserted.

See
International System of Measuring Units
money
pH

specific gravity
units of measure

degrees (°)

Use the symbol with temperatures if the keyboard provides it in reduced-size superscript form; otherwise, spell out *degrees.*

37°C *or* 37 degrees Celsius
98.6°F *or* 98.6 degrees Fahrenheit

Use the degree sign with ECG expressions related to QRS axis. If the symbol is not available, spell out *degrees.*

QRS +60° *or* QRS +60 degrees

Do not use the degree sign with other expressions of degrees, except in mathematical expressions or in tables.

In prone, he does push up to 90 degrees.
not In prone, he does push up to 90°.

See angles

degrees, academic

apostrophe
Use an apostrophe in degree designations such as *master's degree, bachelor's degree,* etc.

capitalization
Use capitals for specific forms and abbreviations, e.g., Bachelor of Arts (BA) degree or Bachelor of Science (BS) degree. Do not capitalize generic forms (bachelor's degree, master's degree). In either case, do not capitalize *degree.*

courtesy titles
When a courtesy title for an academic degree, e.g., *Dr.,* precedes a name, do not use the degree abbreviation after the name. Use one form or the other.

Dr. John Wilson *or* John Wilson, MD *not* Dr. John Wilson, MD

honorary degrees
Omit honorary degree designations.

Barbara Bush *not* Barbara Bush, PhD (hon)

multiple degrees
Use the order preferred by the individual named, separating the degrees by commas. (In the case of publications, such as journals, the publication's editorial style prevails.)
In general, omit academic degrees below the master's level. If an individual has a doctoral degree, omit degrees at master's level or below, unless the master's degree represents a relevant but different or specialized field.

David Bryon, PhD *not* David Bryon, MS, PhD
Stella Jones, MD, MSW

Include specialized professional certifications if pertinent (CMT, RN, PA). Separate multiple degrees (and/or professional credentials) by commas.

Michael Mergener, RPh, PhD
Susan Pierce, CMT, ART

When an individual holds two doctorates, use either or both according to the individual's preference.

Wanda Williams, MD, PhD

periods
While periods continue to be used in academic degrees, the preferred form is without them. If periods are used, do not space within the abbreviation.

Chris Jones, BA *preferred to* Chris Jones, B.A. (*not* B. A.)

salutations and addresses
Use the courtesy title (with last name only) in salutations, the academic title (with full name) in addresses.

Dear Dr. Wilson
John Wilson, MD (*in address*)

signature line
Always use the academic title, never the courtesy title.

Sincerely yours,

John Wilson

John Wilson, MD (*not* Dr. John Wilson)

with names
Place academic degrees after a full name (not just a surname). Place a comma after the full name, then add the degree abbreviation.

John C. Wilson, MD, of Seattle, Washington.

with initials
Do not use degrees or credentials after initials, as in dictator-transcriptionist initials at the end of a report.

JD:DH
not JDMD:DHCMT

See
credentials, professional
titles

degrees, angle
See angles

degrees, burn
See classifications (burn classifications)

degrees, temperature
See temperature, temperature scales

deka-

Inseparable prefix meaning 10 units of a measure. To convert to basic unit, move decimal point one place to the right.

68 dekameters = 680 meters

deoxyribonucleic acid (DNA)

See genetics terminology

department names

See business names

depth

Express with numerals.

4 inches deep

See numbers

derogatory and inflammatory remarks

In general, derogatory or inflammatory remarks do not belong in medical reports except in direct quotations and then only when they are pertinent and essential. Bring their usage in dictation to the attention of the appropriate person, e.g., supervisor, dictator, service owner, client, risk manager, because they may create a risk management situation.

See
editing
risk management

diabetes mellitus terminology

insulin-dependent diabetes, non-insulin-dependent diabetes
References continue to use the hyphens as indicated, and so should medical transcriptionists.

According to the American Diabetes Association (ADA), categories of diabetes include:

type I, IDDM (insulin-dependent diabetes mellitus; previously juvenile-onset): Requires insulin to sustain life.

type II, NIDD (non-insulin-dependent diabetes mellitus; previously adult-onset): Does not require insulin to sustain life. The two subgroups are obese and non-obese.

impaired glucose tolerance: Replaces borderline, chemical, or latent to describe glucose levels between normal and diabetic.

gestational diabetes: Refers to women who develop diabetes during pregnancy; applies only during pregnancy.

diabetes associated with certain conditions or syndromes, e.g., diabetes secondary to endocrine disease.

Classifications of diabetes mellitus in pregnancy include:

class A (gestational diabetes): Transient. *See* gestational diabetes *above.*

class B: Initial onset after age 20, less than 10 years' duration, controlled by diet. Patient may become insulin dependent during pregnancy but not need insulin after delivery.

class C: Onset between ages 10 and 19. Insulin-dependent patient will need increased insulin during pregnancy but will likely return to pre-pregnancy dosage after delivery.

class D: Onset below age 10, with more than 20 years' duration. Patient has hypertension, diabetic retinopathy, and peripheral vascular disease.

class E: Patient has calcification of pelvic vessels.

class F: Patient has diabetic nephropathy.

Infants of diabetic mothers may be described as:

LGA infants: Large for gestational age. Infants of class A, B, and C mothers are apt to be LGA.

SGA infants: Small for gestational age. Infants of class D, E, and F mothers are apt to be SGA.

insulin terminology
Express insulin concentrations as follows:

U100	contains 100 U/mL
U40	contains 40 U/mL
U80	contains 80 U/mL
U500	contains 500 U/mL

Insulin injections are administered intravenously:

preferred term	*also known as*
insulin injection	regular insulin, crystalline zinc
insulin injection, human	regular insulin, human

Insulin suspensions cannot be administered intravenously.

preferred term	*also known as*
insulin suspension, isophane	NPH insulin
insulin suspension, isophane, human	NPH insulin, human
insulin suspension, protamine zinc	PZI
insulin zinc suspension	lente insulin
insulin zinc suspension, extended	ultralente insulin
insulin zinc suspension, prompt	semilente insulin

diacritics, diacritical marks
  See accent marks

Diagnosis, *n. A physician's forecast of disease by the patient's pulse and purse.*
Ambrose Bierce

diagnoses
  Express in full in report sections designating impression, admission diagnosis, discharge diagnosis, preoperative diagnosis, and postoperative diagnosis. Do not abbreviate.
  In headings, when *diagnosis* is dictated, it is preferable (but not required) to change it to the plural form *diagnoses* if more than one is listed.
  When only one diagnosis is given, it is preferable not to number it, even if a number is dictated, because the number gives the appearance that there are additional diagnoses.

DIAGNOSIS
Appendicitis.
preferred to
DIAGNOSIS
1. Appendicitis.

While diagnostic terms must not be abbreviated in statements of diagnoses, descriptive terms relating to the diagnosis may be abbreviated. When measurements are given, use abbreviations for the units of measure.

Retinal tear, OD.
Laceration, 5 mm, left abdomen.

"same"
When "same" is dictated for the discharge diagnosis (meaning same as admission diagnosis) or for the postoperative diagnosis (meaning same as preoperative diagnosis), do not transcribe "same"; repeat the diagnosis in full.

D: Admission diagnosis: Cholelithiasis.
    Discharge diagnosis: Same.
T: Admission diagnosis: Cholelithiasis.
    Discharge diagnosis: Cholelithiasis.

D: Preoperative diagnosis: Uterine fibroid.
    Postoperative diagnosis: Same.
T: Preoperative diagnosis: Uterine fibroid.
    Postoperative diagnosis: Uterine fibroid.

Beware of similar incomplete statements for the names of operations, and transcribe them in full.

D: Repair of same. (*Reference to preoperative diagnosis of left testicular hernia.*)
T: Repair of left testicular hernia.

See
abbreviations
lists

diagonal (/)
Also known as *slash, solidus,* or *virgule.*

See virgule

dictated but not read
Some dictators and/or supervisors request or direct that the statement "dictated but not read" (or a similar phrase such as "transcribed but not read") be entered at the end of some or all reports in an attempt to waive the originator's responsibility to read or review the report and confirm its accuracy prior to authentication (signature).

AAMT advises against the use of either phrase. A patient's report is authenticated when it is signed; the signature represents that the report is accurate in the eyes of the authenticator, i.e., the caregiver. Medical transcriptionists must make every effort to be sure the report is as accurate as they can make it, but the final responsibility and authority lie with the originator.

See
audit trails
authentication
risk management
transcribed but not read

dictator
The person who, by voice, creates the document to be transcribed. Also called *originator* or *author.*

See dictator's style

dictator and transcriptionist initials
See formats

dictator's style
The transcriptionist is responsible for retaining the dictator's style as s/he translates the spoken word to the printed word. Yet, the MT must also edit to assure the record's completeness, correctness, coherence, clarity, and readability. There is a fine line between editing and altering

or tampering, and the transcriptionist must diligently avoid changes that constitute alterations or tampering.

See editing

dictionaries, medical and English
  See references

die of, die from
  Patients (and others) die *of,* not *from,* diseases, disorders, conditions, etc. Edit appropriately.

dieresis accent mark (¨)
  See accent marks

differ, different
  To *differ from* means to be unlike. To *differ with* means to disagree. Also, people and things are *different from* not *different than* one another. Watch usage.

differential blood cell count
  See blood counts

dilation, dilatation
  The two terms have become synonymous in meaning, so that each can mean either the act of expanding or the condition of being expanded, so transcribe as dictated. Likewise, transcribe their verb forms, *dilate* and *dilatate,* as dictated.

  dilation and curettage
  or dilatation and curettage

dimensions

Use a lowercased *x* to express *by* in dimensions. Space before and after the *x*.

The mass was 13 x 2 cm.

directional terms used in anatomy

See anatomic terms

directions

See north, south, east, west

dis-, dys-

Consult an appropriate reference for guidance in determining which prefix is used with which terms. Where either form is acceptable, use the preferred.

disconjugate *preferred to* dysconjugate
disequilibrium
displacement
disproportion
dysarthria
dyscrasia
dyskinesia

discharge summary

One of the basic 4 reports. JCAHO refers to the discharge summary as the clinical summary, which "recapitulates the reason for hospitalization, the significant findings, the procedures performed and treatment rendered, and the condition of the patient on discharge." Abbreviation: DS (no periods).

Typical content headings in a discharge summary include:

admitting diagnosis
history of present illness
pertinent past history (past medical history)
physical examination on discharge
laboratory findings
hospital course

condition on discharge
discharge diagnoses (or final diagnoses)
disposition
prognosis
discharge instructions and medications
followup plans

See
Appendix A, "Sample Reports"
basic 4 reports
formats

disease names
Lowercase disease names except for eponyms forming part of the name.

sickle cell disease
diabetes mellitus
pelvic inflammatory disease
Graves disease
Lyme disease
Parkinson disease
parkinsonism
cushingoid

See
compound modifiers
diagnoses
eponyms

> ***They do certainly give very strange and***
> ***new-fangled names to diseases.***
> Plato

displaced modifiers

See dangling modifiers

distance

Express with numerals.

8 miles

See numbers

ditto marks (")

Do not use ditto marks to indicate "the same"; instead, repeat the term or phrase.

Do not use ditto marks as a symbol for *inches,* except in tables as a space-saving device.

The infant was 22 inches long.
not The infant was 22" long.

division names

See business names

division symbol (÷)

Do not use except in tables and mathematical presentations.

DMD

Abbreviation for *Doctor of Dental Medicine* degree.

See degrees, academic

DNA

Abbreviation for *deoxyribonucleic acid.*

See genetics terminology

DO
Abbreviation for *Doctor of Osteopathy* degree.

See degrees, academic

doctor, physician
The term *doctor* refers to a medical or osteopathic doctor or to someone holding another type of doctoral degree, such as PhD, JD, EdD, DDS, etc. Abbreviation: Dr. *or* Dr (final period is still commonly used, but it may be dropped).
The term *physician* refers to a medical or osteopathic doctor.

See Dr., Dr

documentation trails
See audit trails

dollars and cents
See money

dosage, dose
See drug terminology

double entendres
Words or word combinations, as well as abbreviations and chemical symbols, that have varying meanings depending on context. Avoid them in order to avoid unintentional (and usually inappropriate) humor or derogatory implications.

> ***When I use a word, it means just what***
> ***I choose it to mean—neither more nor less.***
> Lewis Carroll

D: He is complaining of SOB.
T: He is complaining of shortness of breath.

See
editing
risk management

DPM

Abbreviation for *Doctor of Podiatric Medicine* degree.

See degrees, academic

Dr., Dr

Courtesy title for doctors. Use only for earned doctorates (medical or other), not honorary doctorates. The use of an ending period is still preferred, but there is a trend toward dropping it.

Dr. Watson
Dr. C. Everett Koop
not Dr. George Bush

Use *Dr.* not *Doctor* in salutations unless the salutation is directed to more than one doctor. Do not use *Drs.* as plural form in salutations; write out *Doctors* instead.

Dear Dr. Watson:
Dear Doctors Watson and Holmes:

Do not use *Dr.* or *Doctor* when credentials are given.

John Watson, MD
not Dr. John Watson, MD

See
degrees, academic
doctor, physician
titles

*I wonder why ye can always read a doctor's bill
an' ye niver can read his purscription.*
Finley Peter Dunne

drug terminology

dose and dosage
　　Dose means the amount to be administered at one time, or total
amount administered. *Dosage* means regimen and is usually expressed
as a quantity per unit of time.

　　dose:　　5 mg
　　dosage:　5 mg q.i.d.

　　Use lowercased abbreviations with periods for Latin abbreviations
that are related to doses and dosages. Avoid using all capitals because
they draw the eye to the abbreviation rather than to the drug name.
Avoid lowercased abbreviations without periods because some may be
misread as words. Do not translate.

abbreviation	Latin phrase	English translation
a.c.	ante cibum	before meals
b.i.d.	bis in die	twice a day
h.	hora	hour
h.s.	hora somni	at bedtime
n.p.o.	nil per os	nothing by mouth
n.r.	non repetatur	do not repeat
o.d.	omni die	every day
p.c.	post cibum	after meals
p.o.	per os	by mouth
p.r.n.	pro re nata	as needed
q.	quaque	every
q.d.	quaque die	every day
q.h.	quaque hora	every hour
q.i.d.	quarter in die	four times a day
q.4h.	quaque 4 hora	every four hours
t.i.d.	ter in die	three times a day
u.d.	ut dictum	as directed

In expressions that mix Latin abbreviations and English terms, change the English term to a Latin abbreviation, or vice versa.

q.d. *not* q. day
q.4h. *not* q. 4 hours *not* q.4h

Note: AAMT is aware of the keystroke-saving trend toward *bid* and *tid* rather than *b.i.d.* and *t.i.d.* We oppose the trend and continue to discourage dropping periods in lowercased abbreviations that might be misread as words. If you must drop the periods, use all capitals, but keep in mind that AAMT opposes the overuse of capitals, particularly in relation to drug doses and dosages because they draw more attention to the capitalized abbreviations than to the drug names themselves.

Oral dosage forms include pills, tablets, and capsules. Liquid dosage forms may be solutions, emulsions, and suspensions. Topical dosage forms include suspensions or emulsions, such as ointments, creams, lotions, and gels. Other dosage forms include granules, powders, transdermal patches, ocular inserts, suppositories, subdermal pellets, solutions, sprays, drops, and injections.

The most common dosage route is oral for absorption through stomach or intestinal walls. Another common route is parenteral, such as intravenous, intramuscular, subcutaneous, intra-arterial, intradermal, intrathecal, and epidural. Other routes include topical, inhalation, rectal, vaginal, urethral, ocular, nasal, sublingual, and otic.

Do not use commas to separate drug names from doses and instructions. In a series of drugs for each of which the dose and/or instructions are given, use commas to separate each complete entry. Exception: Use semicolons when entries in the series have internal commas.

The patient was discharged on Coumadin 10 mg daily.
The patient was discharged on Carafate 1 g four times daily,
40 minutes after meals and one at bedtime; bethanechol 25 mg
p.o. q.i.d.; and Reglan 5 mg at bedtime on a trial basis.
He was sent home on erythromycin 500 mg q.i.d., Theo-Dur 300 mg
b.i.d., and Tenormin 50 mg q.d.

systems of measurement for drugs
Most pharmaceutical measurements for weight and volume are in the metric system. However, some units from the apothecary and avoirdupois systems remain in use.

apothecary system

weight	liquid measure
1 grain (gr)	1 minim
1 scruple (20 gr)	1 fluidram (60 minims)
1 dram (60 gr)	1 fluidounce (8 fluidrams)
1 ounce (480 gr)	1 pint (16 fluidounces)
1 pound (5760 gr)	1 gallon (4 quarts or 8 pints)

avoirdupois system
1 grain
1 ounce (437.5 grains)
1 pound (16 ounces or 7000 grains)

brand name

The brand name is the same as the trademark or proprietary name. It may suggest a use or indication, and it often incorporates the manufacturer's name. Capitalize brand names. *See* trademark *below.*

Tagamet

code name

The code name is the temporary designation for an as-yet-unnamed drug; it is assigned by the manufacturer. It may include a code number or code designation (number-letter combination).

chemical name

The chemical name describes the chemical structure of a drug. The American Chemical Society, which is the internationally recognized source for such names, follows a set of guidelines established by chemists. Do not capitalize chemical names.

acetylsalicylic acid

generic name

The generic name is also known as the nonproprietary name, the established, official name for a drug. In the United States, it is created by the US Adopted Names Council (USAN). International nomenclature is coordinated by the World Health Organization.

Generic names are in the public domain; their use is unrestricted. Do not capitalize generic names. When the generic name and brand name of a medication sound alike, use the generic spelling unless it is certain that the brand name is being referenced.

aminophylline (generic name) *not* Aminophyllin (brand name)

trademark
The trademark is the manufacturer's name for a drug. Capitalize trademark names. The trademark is also known as the brand name or the proprietary name.

Tagamet

trade name
The trade name is a broader term than trademark, identifying the manufacturer but not the product. Capitalize trade names.

Bayer
Dr. Scholl's

isotope nomenclature
Used in reference to radioactive drugs. Express as indicated below.
When the element name, not the symbol, is used, place the isotope number on-line after the name in the same typeface and type size; do not superscript or subscript. Space between the element name and the isotope number. Do not hyphenate either the noun or the adjectival form.

iodine 128
technetium 99m

When the element symbol is used, place the isotope number as a superscript immediately before the symbol. If superscripts are not available, use the following format: element symbol, space (*not* hyphen), isotope number (on-line), *or* avoid the nonsuperscript form by using the element name followed by the isotope number.

^{128}I or iodine 128
^{99m}Tc or Tc 99m or technetium 99m

For trademarked isotopes, follow the style of the manufacturer. The usual usage in trademarks is for the isotope to be joined to the rest of the name by a hyphen; it may or may not be preceded by the element symbol.

Glofil-125
Hippuran I 131

interferons

A small class of glycoproteins that exert antiviral activity. Use nonproprietary names as discussed below. For trade names and additional guidance, consult the USAN Dictionary or other appropriate reference.

For general classes of compounds or single compounds, follow the lowercased interferon by the spelled-out Greek letter; use the Greek symbol in abbreviations. Note: *alfa* is the correct spelling in these terms, not *alpha*.

interferon alfa	IFN-α
interferon beta	IFN-ß
interferon gamma	IFN-γ

For individual, pure, identifiable compounds with nonproprietary names, add a hyphen, an arabic numeral, and a lowercased letter.

interferon alfa-2a
interferon alfa-2b
interferon gamma-1a
interferon gamma-1b

For names of mixtures of interferons from natural sources, add a hyphen, a lowercased *n,* and an arabic numeral.

interferon alfa-n1
interferon alfa-n2

multiple-drug regimens

Abbreviations for multiple-drug regimens are acceptable if widely used and readily recognized.

MOPP (methotrexate, vincristine sulfate, prednisone, and procarbazine)

vitamins

Lowercase *vitamin,* capitalize the letter designation, and use arabic numerals (in subscript form if available). Do not use a hyphen or space between the letter and numeral.

vitamin B_{12} *or* vitamin B12
B_{12} vitamin *or* B12 vitamin

vitamin	*drug name*
vitamin B_1	thiamine hydrochloride
vitamin B_2	riboflavin
vitamin B_6	pyridoxine hydrochloride
vitamin B_{12}	cyanocobalamin
vitamin C	ascorbic acid
vitamin D_2	ergocalciferol
vitamin D_3	cholecalciferol
vitamin K_1	phytonadione
vitamin K_3	menadione

For additional information on drug terminology, see "Introduction to Pharmaceutical Terminology," by Michael A. Mergener, RPh, PhD, which is Chapter V in the *Introductory Module Handbook* from the *Introductory Module* in AAMT's Exploring Transcription Practices™ series of modules. Contact AAMT for handbook and module prices.

See
chemical nomenclature
International System of Measuring Units
names
units of measure

due to
See because, due to, since

Dukes classification of carcinoma
See cancer classifications

DVM
Abbreviation for *Doctor of Veterinary Medicine* degree.

See degrees, academic

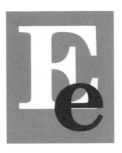

each
> Singular term, so it takes a singular verb.
>
> Each patient was complaining of …
> Each of the tests was repeated x 3.

each other, one another
> Use *each other* when referring to two persons, *one another* for more than two. When the number is indefinite, use either phrase.
>
> Her two physicians kept each other informed about her condition.
> His numerous physicians kept one another informed about his
> > progress.

Earth
> *See* heavenly bodies

earthquake magnitude scale
> *See* scales

east, eastern, East, Eastern
> *See* north, south, east, west

ECG
Preferred to *EKG* as abbreviation for electrocardiogram, electro-cardiography, electrocardiographic.

See cardiology terminology

I am the king of the Romans and above grammar.
Emperor Sigismund I

editing
Verbatim transcription of dictation is seldom possible. Therefore, editing is appropriate in medical transcription when it is done to improve the correctness, clarity, consistency, and completeness of medical dicta-tion—provided it doesn't tamper with the meaning of the report or with the dictator's style.

   D: The patient developed a puffy right eye, which was felt to be secondary to an insect bite by the ophthalmologist.
   T: The patient developed a puffy right eye; this was felt by the ophthalmologist to be secondary to an insect bite.

   D: CAT scan showed there was nothing in the brain but sinusitis.
   T: CAT scan of the brain showed only sinusitis.

MTs should not impose their style on reports, but they should prepare reports that are as correct, clear, consistent, and complete as can be reasonably expected. Tools for editing include dictionaries, word books, style books, textbooks, grammar software, and other teaching materials, experts, and experience.

Editing is inappropriate in medical transcription when it alters information without the editor being certain of the appropriateness or accuracy of the change, when it second-guesses the dictator, when it deletes appropriate and/or essential information, and when it tampers with the dictator's style.

Hospital or department policy and physician preference are major factors in decisions to edit. To the extent that editing is acceptable in your setting and to the dictating physician, the following guidelines for editing are recommended.

Edit grammar, punctuation, spelling, and similar dictation errors as necessary to achieve clear communication. Likewise, edit slang words and phrases, incorrect terms, incomplete phrases, English or medical inconsistencies, and inaccurate phrasing of laboratory data. *See* sections addressing specific areas for additional guidelines and examples.

D: temp
T: temperature

D: Operation: Teflon tube.
T: Operation: Teflon tube insertion.

Transcription departments should provide written instructions to deal with inappropriate language or inflammatory remarks in dictation. Medical transcriptionists should check with their supervisors to determine the rules for editing or omitting such language and remarks from transcription.

Never delete negative or normal findings as dictated. To do so is altering the dictation as well as the medical record.

Use the patient's record to clarify or correct content in dictation. If the record is not available, draw attention to errors or potentially confusing entries for which you do not have sufficient information to make corrections.

Leave a blank space in a report rather than guessing what was meant or transcribing unclear or obviously incorrect dictation. Flag the report to draw attention to the blank and seek the correct information.

> ***No passion in the world is equal to the passion to alter someone else's draft.***
> H.G. Wells

When flagging a report to draw attention to unclear or incorrect dictation, cite the page, section, and line number; place a faint pencil mark in the margin to assist in locating the problem area. If the word or phrase is unfamiliar, note what it sounds like. If the term is inconsistent, briefly state why, e.g., "A left below-knee amputation is later referred to as right BK amputation. Which is correct?"

Similarly, draw attention to medical inconsistencies you have corrected, in order to encourage physician review to assure accuracy.

When transcribing dictation by those who speak English as a second language, edit obvious errors, following the general guidelines for editing. It is not necessary or recommended that such dictation be rewritten; rather, the physician's basic style should be retained.

> *See*
> back-formations
> blank
> coined terms
> derogatory and inflammatory remarks
> dictator's style
> English-as-a-second-language dictators
> errors in dictation
> flag
> grammar
> inconsistencies in dictation
> jargon
> negative findings
> obscenities, profanities, vulgarities
> risk management
> sentences
> slang
> spelling
> verbatim transcription

EEG

Abbreviation for *electroencephalography, electroencephalograph,* and *electroencephalogram.*

> *See* electroencephalographic terms

effect

> *See* affect, effect

e.g.

> *See* Latin abbreviations

either
Replace with *both* unless the meaning is one or the other, *not* both.

Either the left leg or the right leg is involved.

There were wounds on both legs.
not There were wounds on either leg.

either...or, neither...nor
Correlative conjunctions. With an *either...or* or *neither...nor* construction, match the number of the verb with the number of the nearest subject.

Neither the sister nor the brother exhibits similar symptoms.
Neither the sisters nor the brothers exhibit similar symptoms.
Neither the sister nor the brothers exhibit similar symptoms.
Neither the brothers nor the sister exhibits similar symptoms.

EKG
Though still used by some, this is an outdated abbreviation for *electrocardiogram, electrocardiography, electrocardiograph.* The preferred term is *ECG*.

See cardiology terminology

electroencephalographic terms

EEG
Abbreviation for *electroencephalogram, electroencephalography, electroencephalograph.*

symbols for electrodes
Capital letters refer to anatomic areas. Subscript lowercased letters refer to relative electrode positions. Subscript odd numbers refer to electrodes placed on the left, subscript even numbers refer to those on the right, and subscript z refers to midline (zero) electrodes. If subscripts are not available, place the lowercased letters, numbers, and z on-line, adjacent to the capital letter and to each other, or spell out the terms.

A_1, A_2	earlobe electrodes
C_z, C_3, C_4	central electrodes
F_7, F_8	anterior temporal electrodes
F_{pz}, F_{p1}, F_{p2}	frontal pole; prefrontal electrodes
F_z, F_3, F_4	frontal electrodes
O_z, O_1, O_2	occipital electrodes
P_{g1}, P_{g2}	nasopharyngeal electrodes
P_z, P_3, P_4	parietal electrodes
T_3, T_4	midtemporal electrodes
T_5, T_6	posterior temporal electrodes

frequency
Express in cycles per second (c/s *or* cps) or hertz (Hz).

16 c/s *or* 16 cps *or* 16 Hz

some terms commonly used in EEG reports
alert, drowsy, and sleeping states
alpha range
alpha rhythm
alpha waves
amplitude
artifact
background rhythm
beta rhythms
bisynchronous
central sleep spindles
cycles per second (c/s, cps)
delta brush
delta spikes
delta waves
frontal sharp transient
hyperventilation
lambda rhythm
lateralizing focus
mu pattern
occipital driving
paroxysmal, paroxysms
photic stimulation
rhythmic activity
sharp elements
sharp waves
sleep spindles

slow transients
slow waves
spike and dome complex
spike and wave pattern
spikes
spindles
Standard International lead placements
symmetrical activity
synchronous
theta activity
theta frequency
21-channel recording
vertex waves
voltage
wave bursts

*The system treats what is reported to it as real;
the outside reality is immaterial.*
Melvin J. Sykes

electronic monitoring
A process by which electronic means are used to monitor employees
and their output, sometimes jeopardizing the employees' privacy.

See Appendix I, "Electronic Monitoring: Outquotes and Thoughts"

electronic signatures
See Appendix E, "AAMT Position Paper: Providers' Signatures"

ellipsis points (...)
Three dots (periods) used to represent an omission of one or more words.
When the omission occurs at the end of a sentence, the ellipsis points
follow the ending punctuation.

What do you suppose he meant by that remark? ...

If one or more additional sentences are omitted immediately following a sentence ending with ellipses, do not add additional dots.

elliptical construction

One in which one or more words have been left out but are understood. Use a semicolon to separate the elliptical construction from what precedes it; a comma is acceptable if the elliptical construction does not require other internal punctuation.

The white count was abnormal; the red, normal.
or The white count was abnormal, the red normal.

end-of-line word division

AAMT recommends that end-of-line word division be avoided so as to enhance readability.

See word division

ended, ending

Use *ended* to refer to the past, *ending* to refer to the future.

He was seen the week ended June 17.
He will be seen the week ending June 23.

endocrinology terminology

See
diabetes mellitus terminology
hormones

English-as-a-second-language dictators (ESL dictators)

Also known as English-as-a-foreign-language dictators. ESL dictators present special challenges to medical transcriptionists because their pronunciation and sentence structure may be more reflective of their native language than of English. While editing should be minimal, the MT should edit sufficiently for ease of reading and understanding.

See editing

entry-level medical transcriptionist
See medical transcriptionist

enumerations
Enumerations may be horizontal or vertical, depending on their purpose, where they occur in the report, and how they are dictated.

See
lists
outlines
series

> ***Physicians think they do a lot for a patient***
> ***when they give his disease a name.***
> Immanuel Kant

eponyms
A name of a drug, disease, anatomic structure, operation, etc., derived from the name of a person or place. Do not use the possessive form.

Homans sign
Lyme disease

capitalization
Capitalize eponyms but not the common nouns, adjectives, and prefixes that accompany them. Do not capitalize words derived from eponyms.

ligament of Treitz
red Robinson catheter
non-Hodgkin lymphoma
Parkinson disease
Cushing syndrome
but parkinsonism, cushingoid

plurals
Do not use an apostrophe in the plural forms of eponyms.

Babinskis were negative.

possessive form
Do not use the possessive form with eponyms. AAMT adopted this standard because it promotes clarity and consistency. While the use of the possessive form with eponyms remains acceptable, AAMT urges that it be dropped. Our position was discussed at length in the editorial titled "Straight from the Source's Mouth," in the fall 1990 (Vol. 9, No. 3) issue of *JAAMT,* and is reprinted as Appendix J of this book.

AAMT is not alone in promoting the use of eponyms without showing possession. Dr. Edward Huth in *Medical Style & Format* (ISI Press, Philadelphia, 1987, p. 133) wrote that "The time has come to abandon the possessive forms of eponymic terms and simplify usage to nonpossessive form," pointing out that this has been done in *Current Medical Information and Terminology* (American Medical Association, Chicago) since 1971.

In the introduction to the *Dictionary of Medical Eponyms* (The Parthenon Publishing Group, Park Ridge, New Jersey, 1987, p. vi), authors B.G. Firkin and J.A. Whitworth note "we have adopted the suggestion of a number of medical editors by dropping the use of the possessive in eponyms for clarity."

The eighth edition of the *American Medical Association's Manual of Style* (Williams & Wilkins, Baltimore, 1989, p. 251) speaks of "considerable debate over the retention or deletion of the possessive with eponyms," but because of strongly divided feelings "recommends current usage as demonstrated in the most recent editions of *Dorland's* or *Stedman's* medical dictionaries." The AMA stance leads to confusion because of the inconsistencies within and between such learned tomes as the two AMA-cited medical dictionaries, as described below.

The "How to Use This Dictionary" section of the 25th edition of *Stedman's Medical Dictionary* (Williams & Wilkins, Baltimore, 1990, p. xxiii) describes the traditional use and non-use of the possessive form with eponymic terms, observes that the use of the possessive form is "increasingly less common, particularly in certain specialties," then leaves the user to determine the dictionary's preference on a term-by-term basis.

The "Notes on the Use of This Dictionary" section of the 27th edition of *Dorland's Illustrated Medical Dictionary* (W. B. Saunders, 1988, p. xv) likewise admits "the use of the possessive form ending in 's for eponyms is becoming progressively less common," and boldly admits

"The Dictionary...presents an inconsistent mixture of forms, even in the cross references." Finally it warns the user "...the variation in forms in the Dictionary is only a reflection of change and not a prescription for the use of possessive and nonpossessive forms."

Caveat emptor, but which of the inconsistent forms should the medical transcriptionist use? AAMT's answer is clear: Don't be inconsistent. Drop the possessive form with eponyms.

> *See*
> Appendix J, "Straight from the Source's Mouth"
> compound modifiers

equal
Does not have comparative or superlative forms. Thus, *more equal* and *most equal* are incorrect forms. *Equitable* is probably the term intended in such constructions.

A more equitable solution to the problem would be ...
not A more equal solution to the problem would be ...

equal, equal to (=)
Do not use the symbol except in tables and mathematical presentations.

equally
Not *equally as*.

The twins were equally developed.
not The twins were equally as developed.

equator readings
Use a colon to express equator readings.

Sclerotomy drainage was done at the 8:30 equator.

Sometimes, *equator* or a substitute (e.g., *position*) may not be dictated. Add the term if its absence may confuse the reader (who may interpret it as time rather than position).

D: Sclerotomy drainage was done at 8:30.
T: Sclerotomy drainage was done at the 8:30 position.

equipment terms
Capitalize brand (proprietary) names of equipment, and lowercase adjectives and nouns that accompany them. Do not use trademark symbols (™ or ®). Lowercase generic (nonproprietary) names.

American Optical photocoagulator

model numbers
Use arabic numerals to express model numbers of instruments, equipment, etc. Lowercase *model.* Use capital or lowercased letters, the number symbol (#), hyphens, and spaces as they are used by the manufacturer. If not known, use capital letters and no hyphens or spaces, except as dictated.

model C453
model #8546

serial numbers
Use arabic numerals to express serial numbers of instruments, equipment, etc. Lowercase *serial.* Use capital or lowercased letters, the number symbol (#), hyphens, and spaces as they are used by the manufacturer. If not known, use capital letters and no hyphens or spaces, except as dictated.

serial #A185403

See names

errors and omissions insurance
An insurance industry term for professional liability insurance.

See professional liability insurance

errors in dictation
Alertness to errors in dictation is a form of risk management. Medical transcriptionists should watch for and correct obvious errors in dictation, including grammar, spelling, terminology, and style. When uncertain,

draw suspected errors to the attention of the dictator and/or supervisor. Leave a blank and flag it when the change would be significant, particularly if it would influence medical meaning.

See
blank
editing
flag
grammar
risk management

ESL dictators

Abbreviation for *English-as-a-second-language* dictators.

See English-as-a-second-language dictators

esophagram, esophagogram

Esophagogram is the preferred term, but *esophagram* is an acceptable alternative and should be transcribed if dictated.

et al.

See Latin abbreviations

et cetera, etc.

See Latin abbreviations

ex-

Use a hyphen to form *ex-* compounds when *ex-* means former and precedes a noun that can stand on its own. Otherwise, *ex-* is joined directly to the following term (without a hyphen), with the usual exceptions for prefixes applying.

ex-husband
ex-president
excretion
exfoliate

See prefixes

exam

Acceptable brief form of *examination* when dictated, except as a heading.

The physical exam was negative.

PHYSICAL EXAMINATION
Head normal. Neck supple.

Do not use the brief form if not dictated.

D: physical examination
T: physical examination *not* physical exam

Cut out all those exclamation marks.
An exclamation mark is like
laughing at your own joke.
F. Scott Fitzgerald

exclamation mark (!)

Use an exclamation mark to express great surprise, incredulity, or other forceful emotion or comment. Use it primarily in direct quotations; avoid it otherwise except in rare instances. Use a comma or period for mild exclamations.

The patient loudly insisted, "You have already examined me!"
"No," I replied quietly but firmly.

Place the exclamation mark inside the ending quotation mark if the material being quoted is an exclamatory statement. Never combine the exclamatory mark with a period, comma, question mark, or other exclamation mark.

"Stop!" the patient cried as I approached her with the needle and syringe.
not "Stop!," the patient cried as I approached her with the needle and syringe.

The patient insisted, "You have already examined me!"
not The patient insisted, "You have already examined me!".

Place the exclamation point before the closing parenthesis when an exclamatory statement is placed within parentheses.

The patient insisted I had already examined her (I had not!) and refused to cooperate.

Place the exclamatory mark outside the closing parenthesis when the parenthetical matter is not an exclamatory statement but is placed just prior to the end of an exclamatory statement.

What a fiasco (no examination could be done)!

expendable words
Redundant words or phrases that not only can be omitted without changing the meaning, but whose omission improves readability. Avoid overuse and misuse. Examples follow.

it goes without saying
needless to say
in other words
it was shown that
quite
very
rather

For the following phrases, drop the redundant words (those in italics).

12 noon
12 midnight
a.m. *o'clock*
a.m. *in the morning*
at this *point in* time
blood pressure *reading*
consensus *of opinion*
e.g., *for example*
etc., *and so forth*
i.e., *that is*
my *personal* view
p.m. *in the evening*

round *in shape*
small *in size*
sum *total*
two halves
yellow *in color*

**The most valuable of all talents is that of
never using two words when only one will do.**
Thomas Jefferson

exponents
If equipment does not allow superscripting for expressing exponents, use the abbreviations *cu* or *sq* instead. Avoid placing the numerals on-line since the terms are not easily read in this form

4 m^2 *or* 4 sq m *(avoid* m2*)*
8 m^3 *or* 8 cu m *(avoid* m3*)*

See International System of Measuring Units

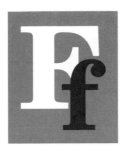

FAB classification

See cancer classifications

factors

See
clotting factor terms
complement factors

Fahrenheit

See temperature, temperature scales

fall

See seasons

false titles

See titles

family relationship names

Capitalize words that denote family relationships only when they are within quotations and they precede the person's name or when they stand alone as a substitute for the name.

Family history: She reported, "My Grandmother Ross raised me."

He said, "Mother told me ..."
but He said his mother told him ...

Otherwise, as when dictator refers to a patient's relative by a familiar term, edit to the formal term.

D: Mom says there was no fever.
T: The patient's mother says there was no fever.

farther, further

Farther refers to physical distance; *further,* to extension of time or degree.

He drove farther than planned.
He needs further care before discharge.

fax

Brief form for *facsimile* or *facsimile machine.* Lowercase is preferred. Do not use periods. Plural: *faxes.* Also a verb: *fax, faxes, faxed, faxing.*

His previous physician faxed the report to me.

February

See months

fellow

Lowercase when referring to academic or specialty position.

He is a fellow of the dermatology board.

fever

See temperature, temperature scales

fewer, less

Fewer refers to a number of individuals or things. *Less* refers to a single amount or mass. Do not use the terms interchangeably.

He has fewer complaints than previously.
He has less pain than previously.

Quantities accompanied by a unit of measure are considered a collective noun, so use *less.*

The lesion was less than 5 mm in diameter.

FIGO staging
See cancer classifications

figure
Numeral or number symbol: 1, 2, 3, 4, 5, 6, etc.

fingerbreadth
Plural form is *fingerbreadths.*

flag
Notation by medical transcriptionist to dictator about a specific report, drawing attention to missing data, unclear dictation, errors in dictation, inconsistent dictation, equipment problems, potentially inflammatory remarks, etc. Flags contribute to risk management.

When flagging a report, cite the page, section, and line number; place a faint pencil mark in the margin to assist in locating the problem area. If the word or phrase is unfamiliar, note what it sounds like. If the term is inconsistent, briefly state why, e.g., "A left below-knee amputation is later referred to as right BK amputation. Which is correct?"

Similarly, flag medical inconsistencies you have corrected, in order to permit physician review to assure accuracy.

See
blank
editing
errors in dictation
inconsistencies in dictation
risk management

fluidounce, fluid ounce
> *See*
> drug terminology
> ounce

followup, follow up
Followup is the preferred noun and adjective form, but the hyphenated form, *follow-up,* remains acceptable. The verb form must be two words: *follow up.*

> The patient did not return for followup.
> In followup visits, she appeared to improve.
> We will follow up with regular return visits.

> ### *A word is not a crystal, transparent and unchanging. It is the skin of living thought.*
> Oliver Wendell Holmes, Jr.

food
> Lowercase most food names.

> baked beans

Capitalize brand names and trademarks but not the nouns or adjectives that accompany them.

> Campbell's baked beans

Capitalize most proper nouns or adjectives used in food names, except when the meaning does not require the proper noun or adjective. The same rule applies to foreign names. Check appropriate references for guidance.

> Boston baked beans
> french fries
> graham crackers

Manhattan cocktail
melba toast

foot

Basic unit of length in measuring system used in United States.
Equal to 12 inches. The metric equivalent is 30.48 cm. To convert to
approximate centimeters, multiply by 30; for exact conversion, multiply
by 30.48. To convert to approximate meters, multiply by 0.3; for exact
conversion, multiply by 0.3048.

5 feet = 150 cm (approximate)
5 feet = 1.5 m (approximate)

Write out; do not use abbreviation (ft.) or symbol (') except in tables.
Express with numerals. Do not use a comma or other punctuation with
units of the same dimension.

10 feet 11 inches
5 pounds 4 ounces

for example

Latin equivalent is *exempli gratia,* abbreviated *e.g.*

See Latin abbreviations

foreign dictators

Dictators for whom English is not their native language. Also known
as English-as-a-second-language dictators and English-as-a-foreign-
language dictators.

See English-as-a-second-language dictators

foreign terms

Do not italicize foreign abbreviations, words, and phrases that have
become part of standard English or medical language usage. Capitalize,
punctuate, and space according to the language's standards. Omit accent
marks except in proper names or where current usage retains them.

in vivo
cul-de-sac
en masse
peau d'orange
i.e.
resume
facade
cooperation
naive

Italicize those that are not in common usage if word processing equipment allows italics; if it does not, use quotation marks.

Do not translate foreign words or abbreviations unless the dictator translates them.

See
accent marks
drug terminology
Latin abbreviations
personal names, nicknames, and initials

formats

While various institutional formats are acceptable, a single standard format is recommended.

Standard sheets without preprinted report headings are preferred because they permit the physician's dictating style to determine the sequence and length of entries, they improve productivity of the medical transcriptionist, and they reduce costs of supplies and production.

Block format is preferred (all lines flush left) for all reports, as well as correspondence, but institutional and client preferences may vary and prevail.

margins

Leave half-inch to one-inch margins, top and bottom, left and right. Ragged-right margins are preferred over right-justified margins, with all lines flush left (block format). To enhance readability, avoid end-of-line hyphenation except for terms with pre-existing hyphens.

paragraphs

Use paragraphs to separate narrative blocks within sections. In general, start new paragraphs as dictated except when such paragraphing is excessive (some dictators start a new paragraph with every sentence or two) or inadequate (some dictators dictate an entire lengthy report in one paragraph).

With 60 staring me in the face, I have developed
inflammation of the sentence structure and
a definite hardening of the paragraphs.
James Thurber

headings and subheadings

Title reports and sections of reports as dictated. Use all capitals for major headings. Avoid underlining because it diminishes readability.

List admitting diagnoses, impressions, discharge diagnoses, preoperative diagnoses, postoperative diagnoses, names of operations, and similar entries vertically. If the dictator numbers some but not all items, be consistent and number all or none. When a single diagnosis is referred to as number one, it is better to delete the number so that the reader is not led to believe that additional entries are missing.

Obvious headings that are not dictated may be inserted, but this is not required. If the dictator moves in and out of sections, insert the information into the appropriate sections (if equipment permits). Otherwise, it may be preferable to omit headings.

Double-space between major sections of reports.

Vertically list subheadings of report sections to assist the reader in identifying particular subsections. Do not line space between subheadings that are listed vertically.

Do not use abbreviations or brief forms in headings except for such widely used and readily recognizable abbreviations as HEENT, if dictated.

Use all capitals for all words in headings and subheadings of medical reports so that the reader can quickly identify pertinent sections by scanning the report.

Use a colon after a heading or subheading in a medical report if the information following the heading or subheading continues on the same line. Do not substitute a hyphen or a dash for a colon following a heading or subheading. Hyphens and dashes in headings and subheadings create visual clutter and reduce readability.

HEENT: Within normal limits.
LUNGS: No rales or rhonchi.
HEART: No murmurs.

Do not use a colon after a heading if the entry following the heading begins on the next line.

PHYSICAL EXAMINATION
Blood pressure 120/90, heart rate 78 and regular.

Capitalize the word following the heading, whether or not a colon follows the heading. Exception: When quantity and unit of measure immediately follow a heading such as *ESTIMATED BLOOD LOSS*, use numerals.

LUNGS: Within normal limits.

ESTIMATED BLOOD LOSS: 10 cc.

signature block
Enter the signature block four lines below the final line of type, flush left. Use dictator's full name. If title is given, place it directly below dictator's name; use initial capitals.

Ruth T. Gross

Ruth T. Gross, MD
Chief of Pediatrics

initials of dictator and transcriptionist at end of transcript
It is common practice to include dictator and transcriptionist initials at the end of each report. When used, enter the initials flush left two lines below last line of type. Use either all capitals or all lowercased letters for both sets of initials, with a colon or virgule between them. Do not use periods. Do not include academic degrees, professional credentials, or titles.

RH:ST *or* rh:st
RH/ST *or* rh/st

continuation pages
When a transcript is longer than one page, enter *continued* at the bottom of each page prior to the last, and repeat the patient's name and

medical record number, the page number, the type and date of report on each continuation page. Additional data may be noted, according to the employer's or client's preference. Do not carry a single line of a report onto a continuation page. Do not allow a continuation page to include only the signature block and the data following it.

See
Appendix A, "Sample Reports"
lists
outlines
series

formula

A formula may include a combination of numbers and symbols. Plural: *formulas.*

See chemical nomenclature

Fort

Abbreviate or spell out in proper names according to common or preferred usage related to entity in question. Of course, spell out and lowercase generic uses.

Fort Collins
Ft. Laramie

fractions

Use numerals for fractional measurements preceding a noun. Join the fraction to the unit of measure with a hyphen.

A $\frac{1}{4}$-inch incision was made.
A $\frac{3}{4}$-pound tumor was removed.
The abdomen shows a 4 $\frac{1}{4}$–inch scar.
The incision was $\frac{1}{4}$- inch long.

Spell out fractional measurements that are less than one when they do not precede a noun.

The tumor weighed three-quarters of a pound.

Place a hyphen between numerator and denominator when neither contains a hyphen.

one-fourth empty
two-thirds full
but one forty-eighth; twenty-three thirty-eighths *or* $^{23}\!/_{38}$

Hyphenate fractions when they are written out and used as adjectives; do not hyphenate those written out and used as nouns.

one-half normal saline
one third of the calf

ages
Use numerals for fractions in ages.

3 ½ years old
3 ½-year-old child

dimensions
Use numerals for fractions in pairs of dimensions.

The wound was 4 ½ x 3 ½ inches.

tables
Use numerals to express fractions in tables.

mixed fractions
If you cannot create reduced-size fractions that can be placed directly following whole numbers, then use the "numeral-virgule-numeral" style, placing a hyphen between the whole number and the fraction.

1 ½ weeks *or* 1-1/2 weeks
3 ½ *or* 3-1/2
5 ½-year-old girl *or* 5-1/2-year-old girl

See
International System of Measuring Units
virgule

fracture classification systems
See classification systems

fracture-dislocation
Note hyphen.

fraternal organizations and service clubs
Capitalize proper names and those designating membership.

Rotary Club
Rotarian

Capitalize formal titles of those holding office when title is used before a name. Lowercase title when it follows a name.

President Donald McDonald
but
Donald McDonald, president

French, french
Capitalize when referring to the country, its people, or its culture.

French-speaking

Do not capitalize such usage as french fries, french door, french cuff.

French Canadian
Do not hyphenate.

French scale
See scales

Friday
See days of the week

fundal height
See obstetrics terminology

fused participle

Result of failure to use the possessive form of a noun or pronoun when it precedes a participle.

D: We are concerned by the *patient failing* to respond to treatment.
T: We are concerned by the *patient's failing* to respond to treatment.

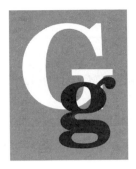

g
Abbreviation for *gram*. Preferred to *gm,* which is still acceptable. Neither form uses a final period.

4 g *preferred to* 4 gm

See gram

gallon
Equal to four quarts or 128 fluidounces. Metric equivalent is approximately 3.8 liters. To convert to liters, multiply by 3.8. Do not abbreviate (*gal*) except in tables.

4 gallons = 15.2 liters

gay
Popular term for a homosexual person, whether male or female. Do not capitalize. Noun and adjective forms are the same.

generic terms
See names

genetics terminology

chromosomal terms
The following discussion of chromosomal terms is adapted from "Some Basics of Genetics and Chromosomal Terminology," by Claudia

Crickmore, CMT, published in *Neonatology Word Book,* by Hazel Tank, CMT, and Catherine Gilliam, CMT, 1991, AAMT. (For price information, contact AAMT.)

There are 46 chromosomes in human cells, occurring in pairs and numbered 1 through 22, plus the sex chromosomes, an X and a Y in males, two X's in females. The non-sex chromosomes are also called autosomes.

group designations: Refer to chromosomes by number or by group.

chromosome	*group*
1-3	A
4, 5	B
6-12, X	C
13-15	D
16-18	E
19, 20	F
21, 22, Y	G

chromosome 16
a chromosome in group E
a group-E chromosome

trisomy: An extra chromosome in any one of the autosomes or of either sex chromosome.

trisomy D: extra chromosome in a group D chromosome, either the 13th, 14th, or 15th chromosome

trisomy 21: an extra 21st chromosome (Down syndrome)

A plus or minus in front of the chromosome number means there is either an extra chromosome or an absent chromosome within that pair.

trisomy 21 = female karyotype: 47,XX +21

The plus or minus following the chromosome number means that part of the chromosome is either extra or missing.

cri du chat syndrome = male karyotype: 46,X6 5p-

arms: Each chromosome has a short arm and a long arm. The short arm is designated by a *p,* the long arm by a *q,* immediately following the chromosome number (no space between). Each arm is divided into regions (from 1 to 4); place the region number immediately following the arm designation. Regions are divided into bands, again joined without a space. If a subdivision is identified, it follows a decimal point placed immediately after the band number.

20p	20th chromosome, short arm
20p1	20th chromosome, short arm, region 1
20p11	20th chromosome, short arm, region 1, band 1
20p11.23	20th chromosome, short arm, region 1, band 1, subdivision 23

A translocation occurs when a segment normally found in a certain arm of a certain chromosome appears in a different location; it may be written as a small *t* with the *from* and *to* sites in parentheses, e.g., t(14q21q), meaning from long arm of 14 to long arm of 21. A more complex designation such as t(2;6)(q34;p12) means from region 3 band 4 of the long arm of chromosome 2 to region 1 band 2 of the short arm of chromosome 6. The chromosome numbers appear in a separate set of parentheses from the arm, region, and band information.

> *Heredity is nothing but stored environment.*
> Luther Burbank

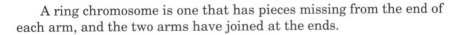

A ring chromosome is one that has pieces missing from the end of each arm, and the two arms have joined at the ends.

bands: Use capital letters to refer to chromosome bands, which are elicited by special staining methods.

band	*stain*
C bands *or* C-banding	constitutive heterochromatin
G bands *or* G-banding	Giemsa
N bands *or* N-banding	nucleolar organizing region
Q bands *or* Q-banding	quinacrine
R bands *or* R-banding	reverse-Giemsa

karyotype: Describes an individual's chromosome complement: the number of chromosomes plus the sex chromosomes present in that individual. Place a comma (without spacing) between the chromosome number and the sex chromosome. Use a virgule to indicate more than one karyotype in an individual.

normal human karyotypes: 46,XX (female)
                            46,XY (male)

some abnormal karyotypes: 47,XXY
                            45,X0
                            48,XXX
                            45,X/46,XX

genes

Molecular units of heredity; their locations are called loci. A gene's main form and its locus have the same symbol, usually an abbreviation for the gene name or a quality of the gene. The symbol usually consists of 3 or 4 characters, all capitals, or all capitals and an arabic number, all on-line (no superscripts or subscripts). Do not use hyphens or spaces. Italics are preferred, but plain type may be used in medical transcription.

CF or CF   cystic fibrosis
G6PD or G6PD   glucose-6-phosphate dehydrogenase
HPRT or HPRT   hypoxanthine phosphoriboxyltransferase
PHP or PHP   panhypopituitarism

Alleles are alternative forms of genes. To express their symbols, add an asterisk and the allele designation to the gene symbol. Italics are preferred, but plain type may be used in medical transcription.

HBB*6V or HBB*6V

biochemical constituents

The biochemical constituents of genetics include deoxyribonucleic acid (DNA), ribonucleic acid (RNA), and the amino acids.

deoxyribonucleic acid (DNA): Includes the bases thymine, cytosine, adenine, and guanine. DNA contains the genetic code and is found in the chromosomes of humans and animals. DNA expressions and their abbreviations include:

complementary DNA	cDNA
double-stranded DNA	dsDNA
single-stranded DNA	ssDNA

ribonucleic acid (RNA): Includes the bases cytosine, adenine, and guanine, and the base uracil (U). RNA is functionally associated with DNA. RNA expressions and their abbreviations include:

heterogeneous RNA	hnRNA
messenger RNA	mRNA
ribosomal RNA	rRNA
small nuclear RNA	snRNA
transfer RNA	tRNA

amino acids of proteins: Write out in text. In tables, use three-letter or one-letter abbreviations.

phenylalanine	Phe	F
proline	Pro	P
tryptophan	Trp	W

oncogenes
Viral genes in certain retroviruses. Express as three-letter lowercased terms derived from names of associated viruses. Italics are preferred, but plain type may be used in medical transcription.

abl or abl
mos or mos
sis or sis
src or src

The prefix *v-* (virus) or *c-* (cellular or chromosomal counterpart) indicates the location of the oncogene. The *c-* prefixed oncogenes are also known as proto-oncogenes and may be alternatively expressed in all capitals, without the prefix. Italics are preferred, but plain type may be used in medical transcription. Note: The prefix is never italicized.

ras or ras
H-*ras or* H-ras

genus and species names

genus
    Includes species whose broad features are alike in organization but
different in detail. Capitalize genus names and their abbreviated forms,
but do not capitalize their plural or adjectival forms. Italics are not preferred in medical transcription.

    Staphylococcus
    staphylococci
    staphylococcal

species
    Group of individuals that can interbreed and produce fertile offspring.
Usually preceded by genus name. Lowercase species names. Italics are
not preferred in medical transcription.

    Homo sapiens
    Escherichia coli
    Staphylococcus aureus

abbreviations
    In second reference to a genus-species term, the genus name may be
abbreviated as a single letter (without a period, according to the *AMA
Manual of Style,* but other references, including *Stedman's / Bergey's
Bacteria Words,* retain the period). A longer abbreviation (again, with
or without a period, depending on reference) may be used to avoid confusion. Do not abbreviate the species name even if the genus name is
abbreviated.

    S aureus *or* S. aureus
    or Staph aureus *or* Staph. aureus

    D: H. flu
    T: H. influenzae

Do not abbreviate a genus name when it stands alone.

    D: coagulase-positive Staph
    T: coagulase-positive Staphylococcus

-osis, -iasis

The suffixes *-osis* and *-iasis* indicate disease caused by a particular class of infectious agents or types of infection. Do not capitalize terms formed with these suffixes.

amebiasis
dermatophytosis

geographic names

abbreviations

Do not abbreviate names of states, territories, countries or similar units within reports when they stand alone. State or territory names may be abbreviated when they are preceded by a city name, and country names may be abbreviated when preceded by a city or state/territory name. Of course, abbreviations may be used in addresses.

capitalization

Capitalize names of political divisions such as streets, cities, towns, counties, states, countries; and topographic names, e.g., mountains, rivers, oceans, islands; and accepted designations for regions.

Wallingford Avenue
Lake Wobegon
Great Britain
the Bay Area
Yosemite National Park
the Middle East

Capitalize common nouns that are an official part of a proper name; lowercase them when they stand alone.

Philippine Islands
the islands

Capitalize compass directions when they are part of the geographic name. *See* north, south, east, west

West Germany

Capitalize geographic names used as eponyms.

Lyme disease

Do not capitalize words derived from geographic names when they have a special meaning.

india ink
plaster of paris
french fries

foreign places
Use primary spelling in recognized English dictionary.

commas
In text, use a comma before and after the state name preceded by a city name, or a country name preceded by a state or city name.

The patient is from San Francisco and moved to Modesto, California, 15 years ago.
The patient returned from a business trip to Paris, France, the week prior to admission.

hyphens
Some combinations of proper adjectives derived from geographic entities are hyphenated; some are not. Some which are not hyphenated in their noun form are hyphenated in their adjectival form. Check appropriate references.

French Canadian
African American *or* African-American

See
Appendix CC, "State Names and Abbreviations, Major Cities, and State/City Resident Designations"
Canada
eponyms
north, south, east, west
state, county, city, and town names and resident designations
street names and numbers
United States
USPS guidelines

giga-
Prefix meaning 1 billion units of a measure. To convert to basic unit, move decimal point nine places to the right (adding zeros as necessary).

8.8 gigatons = 8,800,000,000 tons.

girl
See age referents

Glasgow coma scale
See scales

Gleason score, Gleason tumor grade
See cancer classifications

globulins
Use Greek letters and arabic numerals. Subscript the numerals if equipment permits; otherwise place on-line. If Greek letters are not available, use English translations. Place a hyphen between the Greek letter (with or without subscript) and *globulin* but not between the English translation and *globulin*. Do not subscript the numeral with the English translation; rather, connect it by a hyphen.

ß-globulin
beta globulin
ß$_2$-globulin
beta-2 globulin

immunoglobulins
Express as follows:

IgG
IgM
IgA
IgD
IgE

See Greek letters

gm

Alternative abbreviation for *gram,* but *g* is preferred. Neither form takes a final period.

4 g *preferred to* 4 gm

See gram

government

Always lowercase this term.

federal government
US government
Canadian government
taxes paid to the government

governmental bodies

Capitalize full proper names of governmental agencies, departments, and offices.

the US House of Representatives
the US Supreme Court

Use capitals in shortened versions if the context makes the name of the nation, state, province, etc., clear.

the House of Representatives
Parliament

Lowercase the plural forms of terms such as *Senate, House of Representatives,* that are capitalized in proper names.

California Senate and New York Senate
but California and New York senates

GPA terminology

See obstetrics terminology

gr
Abbreviation for *grain.* Do not confuse with *g* or *gm,* which are abbreviations for *gram.*

See grain

grade
Do not capitalize. Use arabic numerals.

See
cancer classifications
cardiology terminology
GVHD grading system

grain
Smallest unit in US system of weights. Weight of one grain of wheat. There are 437.5 grains in an ounce, 7000 grains in a pound. Abbreviation: gr (no period).

gram
Basic unit of weight in metric system. Approximately one twenty-eighth of an ounce. Multiply by 0.035 to convert to ounces. Abbreviation: *g* is preferred to *gm* (not *gr,* which is abbreviation for *grain*).

grammar
The medical transcriptionist should correct the dictator's obvious grammatical errors.

grammar software
Software that automatically checks the grammar of a document. Grammar software is a supplement to, not a replacement for, the medical transcriptionist's responsibility to proofread documents and assure the accuracy of the grammar within them. Some grammatical errors will pass the scrutiny of software.

See
editing
errors in dictation
proofreading

It is said that one machine can do the work of fifty ordinary men. No machine, however, can do the work of one extraordinary man.
Tehyi Hsieh

grave accent mark(`)
See accent marks

gravida
See obstetrics terminology

gray (Gy)
The International System unit of absorbed dose of ionizing radiation. Equal to one joule per kilogram of tissue. Abbreviation: Gy (no period).

See International System of Measuring Units

greater
Do not use *greater* in place of *more* or *longer.* Edit appropriately.

D: The pain persisted greater than 24 hours.
T: The pain persisted longer than 24 hours.
or The pain persisted more than 24 hours.

Capitalize *greater* when referring to a community and its surrounding area. Lowercase otherwise.

Greater Boston
Greater Los Angeles
the greater metropolitan area

greater than (>)
Do not use the symbol except in formulas and tables.

Greek letters

Spell out the English translation when the word stands alone. Do not capitalize English translations. Use the Greek letter or spell it out when it is part of an extended term, according to the preferred form; consult appropriate references for guidance. In extended terms, use a hyphen after the Greek letter but not after the English translation.

alpha
beta
delta
ß-globulin
beta globulin

See globulins

GVHD grading system

Abbreviation means **g**raft-**v**ersus-**h**ost **d**isease. Use arabic numerals 1 (mild) through 4 (severe), placed on-line directly after the abbreviation (no space). May also be expressed as clinical grade 1 through 4.

GVHD1 *or* GVHD clinical grade 1
GVHD2 *or* GVHD clinical grade 2
GVHD3 *or* GVHD clinical grade 3
GVHD4 *or* GVHD clinical grade 4

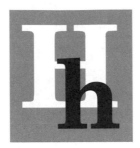

h, h.

Letter *h* (no period) is abbreviation for *hour;* do not use except in virgule constructions and in tables.

40 mm/h
The procedure lasted 1 hour 15 minutes.

Letter *h.* (with period) is abbreviation for Latin *hora,* meaning hour.

q.6h. (every six hours)

In instructions for medications, when Latin abbreviations are coupled with English terms, such as hour, convert English term to Latin abbreviation or vice versa; do not use English abbreviation.

q.4h. *or* every 4 hours *not* q.4 hours *or* q.4h

See drug terminology

Harvard criteria for brain death

In addition to body temperature equal to or higher than 32°C and the absence of central nervous system depressants, all of the following criteria must be met in order to establish brain death.

- unreceptivity and unresponsiveness
- no movement or breathing
- no reflexes
- flat electroencephalogram (confirmatory)

HCFA
Abbreviation for *Health Care Financing Administration,* a bureau of the US Department of Health and Human Services (HHS), which administers federal Medicare and Medicaid programs.

headings and subheadings
See formats

Health Care Financing Administration
See HCFA

heart sounds and murmurs
See cardiology terminology

heavenly bodies

planets, stars, constellations
Capitalize proper names of planets (including Earth), stars, and constellations. Lowercase nouns and adjectives derived from them. Lowercase *sun* and *moon.* Lowercase *earth* when not used as a proper name.

Milky Way
Venus
Earth, earth
lunar
martian

comets
Capitalize the proper name but lowercase *comet.*

Kahoutek comet

hecto-
Inseparable prefix denoting 100 units of a measure. Use *hect-* before a vowel, *hecto-* before a consonant. To convert to basic unit, move decimal point two places to right, adding zeros as necessary.

3.3 hectometers = 330 meters.

height
    Express with numerals, as follows. Write out nonmetric units of measure. Note there is no comma after *feet.*

    Height: 5 feet 8 inches.

    See numbers

hepatitis nomenclature
    Use capital letters to designate type. Do not connect the letter by a hyphen to *hepatitis,* but do use a hyphen to connect *non* to the letter.

    hepatitis A
    hepatitis B
    hepatitis C
    non-A hepatitis
    non-B hepatitis
    delta hepatitis

    related abbreviations

HAV	hepatitis A virus
HBAg	hepatitis B antigen
HBIG	hepatitis B immunoglobulin
HBV	hepatitis B virus
anti-HAV	antibody to HAV
anti-HBV	antibody to HBV

    Previous designations of viral hepatitis, such as infectious hepatitis, short-incubation-period hepatitis, long-incubation-period hepatitis, and serum hepatitis are no longer preferred but should be transcribed if dictated.

hertz
    International unit of frequency equivalent to one cycle per second. Abbreviation: Hz (no period).

his, her
    See sexist language

Hispanic

Adjective referring to US citizen or resident of Latin-American or Spanish descent. *Latino* is also widely used, and *Mexican-American* may be preferred by those of Mexican descent.

See
Latino
Mexican-American
sociocultural designations

historic periods and events

Capitalize widely recognized names for events in history, geology, archeology, anthropology and for historic periods and events.

the Middle Ages
the Vietnam War

Capitalize only proper nouns and adjectives in generic descriptions of periods and events.

ancient Greece

Lowercase references to centuries.

18th century

See years, decades, centuries

historic present

See verbs

history and physical examination

One of the basic 4 reports. Abbreviation: H&P (no periods). Typical content headings in a history and physical include the following.

chief complaint (*or* reason for admission)
history of present illness
past history (past medical history)
social history
family history

review of systems
admission laboratory data
physical examination
admitting diagnosis (*or* impression)
plan

See
Appendix A, "Sample Reports"
basic 4 reports
formats

> *Nowadays, the clinical history too*
> *often weighs more than the man.*
> Martin H. Fisher

HLA
Abbreviation for *human leukocyte antigen.*

See human leukocyte antigens

holidays and holy days
Capitalize the names of secular and religious holidays.

Fourth of July
Memorial Day
Martin Luther King Day
Ascension Sunday
Easter

hopefully
Hopefully means in a hopeful manner.

They waited hopefully for news of his recovery.

Strictly speaking, *hopefully* should not be used to mean *I hope, we hope, it is hoped, let us hope*. However, it is so widely used in this sense that such use is increasingly acceptable. Transcribe such usage if dictated.

Hopefully, his symptoms will respond to the treatment.

horizontal series

See
lists
series

hormones

Hormones may be referred to by their therapeutic or diagnostic names, their native names, or their abbreviations. Use subscripted numerals with abbreviations for thyroxine and triiodothyronine, if subscripting is available; otherwise, place them on-line.

therapeutic/diagnostic name	*native name*	*abbreviation*
chorionic gonadotropin	human chorionic gonadotropin	HCG
corticotropin, purified	corticotropin (previously adrenocorticotropic hormone)	ACTH
triiodothyronine	triiodothyronine	T_3 *or* T3
thyrotropin	thyroid-stimulating hormone	TSH
thyroxine	thyroxine	T_4 *or* T4

The preferred suffix is *-tropin* (indicating an ability to change or redirect), not *-trophic* (indicating a relationship to nutrition).

thyrotropin-releasing hormone
gonadotropin-releasing hormone
corticotropin
somatotropin

however

as an adverb
However may be used to modify one or more adjectives.

However resistant she may be, I will continue to advise her to quit smoking.

as a conjunctive adverb

Place a semicolon before and a comma after *however* when it is used to connect two complete thoughts separated by a semicolon.

He is improved; however, he cannot be released.

Place a comma after *however,* when it serves as a bridge between two sentences separated by ending punctuation.

He is improved. However, he cannot be released.

as an interruptive

When *however* occurs elsewhere in the second sentence (not as its first word), it is called an interruptive and requires a comma before and a comma after it.

He is improved. He cannot, however, be released.

There is disagreement among grammarians as to the best placement of this type of *however.* In medical transcription, place it as dictated provided such placement does not interfere with communication.

D&T: He is improved. He cannot, however, be released.
D&T: He is improved. He cannot be released, however.

See conjunctions

h.s.

See drug terminology

human leukocyte antigens

Express with capital-lowercased combinations and hyphens. Check appropriate references for guidance.

major histocompatibility complex, class I antigens

HLA-A
HLA-B
HLA-C

major histocompatibility complex, class II antigens
HLA-D
HLA-DR

examples of antigenic specificities of major HLA loci
HLA-B27
HLA-DRw10

-hundreds

Numerals are preferred to words.

1900s *not* nineteen-hundreds

Hunt and Hess neurological classification

See classifications

> ### *If you take hyphens seriously*
> ### *you will surely go mad.*
> John Benbow

hyphens

Hyphens as word connectors or joiners may be permanent or temporary. Over time, hyphenated terms may be replaced with the solid form. Check appropriate references for guidance.

Do not space before or after a hyphen. Exception: Single-space after a suspensive hyphen (one used to connect a series of compound modifiers with the same base term).

We used 3- and 4-inch bandages.

clarity

Use hyphens to avoid confusion in meaning.

re-create (make again) *not* recreate (play)
re-cover (cover again) *not* recover (from illness)

Use hyphens to assist in pronunciation.

co-workers
re-study

vowel strings
Sometimes, use a hyphen to break up a string of three or more vowels, but sometimes do not.

ileo-ascending
but radioactive

missing letters or numbers
Use a double hyphen or em dash to represent missing letters or numbers. Be sure to place a space after the em dash or double hyphen used to represent the ending letters or numbers in a term.

What the h— did he think I would do?

telephone numbers
Use a hyphen or en dash following the area code and prefix of a telephone number.

209-551-9317
209–551–9317

ZIP codes
Use a hyphen or en dash between the first five and last four digits of a ZIP-plus-four code.

Modesto, CA 95357-6187
Modesto, CA 95357–6317

Use appropriate references to determine hyphenation of terms not covered by these guidelines or the following cross-references.

See specific topics, including
compound modifiers
compound words
dashes
fractions
letters
numbers
prefixes
range
status post
suffixes
suture sizes
units of measure
vertebra
word division

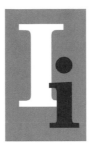

-ible
> *See* -able, -ible

identical
> Follow by either *with* or *to*.
>
> The symptoms are identical with (*or* to) those he exhibited on his last admission.

i.e.
> *See* Latin abbreviations

immunoglobulins
> *See* globulins

Inc.
> *See* business names

inch
> One-twelfth of a foot. Metric equivalent: 2.54 centimeters. Multiply by 2.54 to convert to centimeters.
>
> Write out; do not use abbreviation (*in.*) or symbol (") except in tables. Express with numerals. Do not use a comma or other punctuation between units of the same dimension, i.e., feet and inches.
>
> 12 feet 10 inches

incomparable words

Absolute adjectives that do not have a comparative or superlative form. They include the following.

complete
dead
fatal
pregnant
total
unanimous
unique

Forms such as *more complete* or *slightly pregnant* or *fatally dead* are inappropriate. Terms such as *almost* or *nearly* are, however, acceptable.

almost fatal
nearly total

> *I wouldn't touch a superlative*
> *again with an umbrella.*
> Dorothy Parker

inconsistencies in dictation

When the medical transcriptionist identifies an inconsistency in dictation, s/he should resolve it if this can be done with competence and confidence. If the discrepancy cannot be resolved with certainty, the report should be flagged and brought to the attention of the supervisor or dictator for resolution.

This 45-year-old male is status post hysterectomy. *(Either the patient is not male or he is status post another type of surgery.)*

See
editing
flag
risk management

The whole end of speech is to be understood.
Confucius

infant
> *See* age referents

inflammatory remarks
> *See* derogatory and inflammatory remarks

initialisms
> *See* acronyms

initials

at end of transcript
> *See* format

in names
> *See* personal names, nicknames, and initials

-in-law
> Use hyphens. Plural form: Make primary noun plural; do not add *s* to *law*. Possessive form: Use *'s* after *-law*.

> sister-in-law
> sisters-in-law
> sister-in-law's
> sisters-in-law's

institutions
> *See* business names

insulin-dependent diabetes
See diabetes mellitus terminology

insulin terminology
See diabetes mellitus terminology

interferons
See drug terminology

International System of Measuring Units (SI)

The International System of Units (Système International d'Unités; abbreviated SI) is the system of metric measurements adopted in 1960 at the Eleventh General Conference on Weights and Measures of the International Organization for Standards. Since the 1977 recommendation of the 30th World Health Assembly that SI units be used in medicine, some medical journals use it to a limited degree, some use it only in conjunction with conventional units, and some have not yet adopted it.

Major characteristics of the SI are decimals, a system of prefixes, and a standard defined as an invariable physical measure.

The adoption of SI in the documentation of patient care is likewise sporadic, but it is sufficiently widespread, in whole or in part, to warrant the attention of medical transcriptionists.

basic units and properties of the SI

base unit	*SI symbol*	*basic property*
meter	m	length
kilogram	kg	mass
second	s	time
ampere	A	electric current
kelvin	K	thermodynamic temperature
candela	cd	luminous intensity
mole	mol	amount of substance

units derived from SI's basic units

derived unit	*name and symbol*	*basic unit derived from*
area	square meter (m^2)	meter
volume	cubic meter (m^3)	meter
frequency	hertz (Hz)	second

work, energy	joule (J)	kilogram
pressure	pascal (Pa)	kilogram
force	newton (N)	kilogram
density	kilogram per cubic meter (kg/m^3)	kilogram

prefixes and symbols

The SI combines prefixes with the basic units to express multiples and submultiples of those units. Factors are powers of 10. Note that the SI refers to shortened forms of measure as symbols, not abbreviations.

factor	*prefix*	*symbol*
10^{24}	yotta-	
10^{21}	zetta-	
10^{18}	exa-	E
10^{15}	peta-	P
10^{12}	tera-	T
10^{9}	giga-	G
10^{6}	mega-	M
10^{3}	kilo-	k
10^{-3}	milli-	m
10^{-6}	micro-	μ
10^{-9}	nano-	n
10^{-12}	pico-	p
10^{-15}	femto-	f
10^{-18}	atto-	a
10^{-21}	zepto-	
10^{-24}	yoctu-	

According to the *AMA Manual of Style,* exponents that are multiples of 3 are recommended, and those prefixes that are not multiples of 3 (e.g., *hecto-, deca-, deci-,* and *centi-*) are to be avoided in scientific writing. That avoidance obviously does not extend to patient records, as evidenced by MTs' frequent encounters with the prefix *centi-* (centimeter, centigrade, centigray) and occasional encounters with *deci-* (decigram, deciliter). In general, medical transcriptionists should apply the following rules and guidelines for the SI, but this is not always possible. Exceptions to the following SI rules and guidelines that are necessary, logical, or commonly accepted in medical transcription are noted.

abbreviations

Abbreviate most units of measure accompanying numerals and all those in virgule constructions. Use the same abbreviation for singular and plural forms. Do not use periods with abbreviated units of measure.

1 g
20 g
40 mm/h

area, volume, and magnification
The SI uses the multiplication sign in expressions of area, volume, and magnification. In medical transcription, use a lowercased *x* instead. Space before and after the *x* to enhance readability.

2 x 2-mm area
x 20,000 magnification

commas
Drop the comma in numbers of four digits. In numbers of five or more digits, the SI replaces the comma with a half space. This is not always possible in medical transcription, nor is it commonly seen in patient records, so the continued use of the comma is acceptable and preferred in numbers of five or more digits in medical transcription. But do conform to the SI rule eliminating both the comma and the half space in numbers that contain decimal points.

1234
12,345
12345.67

decimals v fractions
Use the decimal form of numbers when a fraction is given with an abbreviated unit of measure or for a precise measurement. Use mixed fractions for approximate measurements; these usually represent time.

4.5 mm
$5^1/_2$ days
$3^3/_4$ hours

drug dosages
It is expected that all drug dosages will eventually be expressed in SI units. Meanwhile, transcribe the dictated units; do not convert.

exponents
Express exponents, which are preferred to the abbreviations *cu* and *sq,* as superscripts in reduced point size. When equipment does not

readily allow such superscripts, the abbreviations *cu* and *sq* are accept-able. Do not place the exponent numerals on-line in these expressions as they are not easily read when expressed in this manner.

3 m^2 *or* 3 sq m (not *m2*)
9 m^3 *or* 9 cu m (not *m3*)

kelvin v Celsius
    The SI unit for thermodynamic temperature is the kelvin, but the medical transcriptionist is more apt to encounter temperatures reported in degrees Celsius or degrees Fahrenheit. Transcribe the system dictated; do not convert.

numerals
    Use arabic numerals for all quantities with units of measure. Place a space between the numeral and the symbol for the unit of measure. Exceptions: Do not place a space between the numeral and the percent sign, the degree sign, or the Celsius (or Fahrenheit) symbol. Place the quantity and the unit of measure on the same line of type; do not allow one line of type to end with the quantity and the next line to begin with the unit of measure.

48 kg
13.5 mm
48%
40°C

    When a number and unit of measure begin a sentence, write out both the number and unit of measure. In medical transcription, there is the option of recasting the sentence so as to avoid beginning it with a numeral and unit of measure.

Twenty milliequivalents of KCl was given.
KCl 20 mEq was given.

percentage values
    According to the SI, it is common and acceptable for percentage values to be expressed as a fraction of one. MT experience would indi-cate that it is more common and acceptable for *percent* to be dropped in dictation (and thus in transcription). Use the expression dictated. Do not convert unless the forms are mixed; then make them consistent.

polys 58% *or* polys 0.58 *or* polys 58
MCHC 34% *or* MCHC 0.34 *or* MCHC 34

rad v *gray; calorie* v *joule*
    The SI converts *rad* to *gray* (Gy) and *calorie* to *joule.* Transcribe as dictated; do not make the conversion unless directed to do so.

units of time and time abbreviations
    Do not abbreviate expressions of English units of time except in virgule constructions. Do not use periods with such abbreviations. Note: In pharmaceutical expressions (q.h., q.i.d., etc.), the terms are Latin (h., hora; d., die) and take periods, and so the above rule against periods does not apply.

minute	min
week	wk
month	mo
hour	h
day	d
year	y

The patient is 5 days old.
He will return in one week for followup.
40 mm/h
q.4h.

    Efforts have been made here to extract the basic applications of SI rules and guidelines to medical transcription. As indicated, SI usage affects or is affected by many other areas of medical transcription style and practices: grammar, abbreviations, numerals, punctuation, plurals, etc.
    More detail about the SI and SI units is available from the *AMA Manual of Style,* from which much of the above information was drawn, but we caution you that the AMA text speaks to the preparation of medical manuscripts for publication and does not address the preparation of medical reports, i.e., the communication of patient information through medical dictation and transcription. As indicated, some of the differences are pronounced.

    See
abbreviations
decimals, decimal units
fractions

numbers
percent
temperature, temperature scales
time

intervertebral disk space
    See vertebra

isotope nomenclature
    See drug terminology

italics
    Italicized type is more difficult to read than regular type, so it should be used sparingly in medical transcription, avoiding it even in some instances when such usage would be required elsewhere, e.g., in manuscripts. Use the following guidelines.

abbreviations
    Do not italicize.

allergies
    Do not italicize. *See* allergies

arbitrary designations
    Do not italicize letters used for arbitrary designations.

    brand X
    subject A

chemical elements and compounds
    Do not italicize symbols for chemical elements and compounds.

    KCl

foreign institutions and organizations
    Do not italicize names of foreign institutions and organizations.

foreign words or phrases
    Do not italicize terms that are commonly used in the English or medical language.

in toto
cul-de-sac
en masse
peau d'orange
bruit

genus and species
It is acceptable but neither preferred nor necessary to italicize Latin names for genera and species in patient records. Regular type is preferred.

Staphylococcus aureus

letters referred to as letters
Use italics. If not available, use quotation marks.

Use a capital *C* in the term Celsius.

letters indicating shape
Do not italicize letters indicating shape.

I beam
Z incision

letters in musical notation
Do not italicize letters indicating musical notations.

B minor
C clef

irony, slang, coined expressions, inexact usage, or unusual usage
Do not italicize. Use quotation marks instead.

an "impatient" patient
not an *impatient* patient

titles of books, periodicals, plays, films, long poems, paintings, sculptures, and legal case titles in text
Use italics. If not available, underline.

The patient is the author of *The Surgical Word Book*.

words referred to as words
Use italics. If not available, use quotation marks.

It's is the contraction for *it is.*

See regular type

it's, its
Do not confuse or misuse these soundalikes.

it's
Contraction for *it is.* Remember that contractions are not appropriate in medical reports except in direct quotes.

It's time to go.

its
Possessive form of *it.*

its dimensions

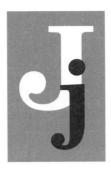

Jaeger eye chart

Pronounced *yaeger.* A *J* followed by an on-line arabic number specifies the line with the smallest letters that the patient can read. Do not space between the letter and number.

J5

January

See months

Incomprehensible jargon is
the hallmark of a profession.
Kingman Brewster

jargon

Cliches of a profession are referred to as jargon. Medical jargon tends to be particularly imprecise and may be offensive or derogatory. In general, avoid its use by rephrasing.

D: urines
T: urine samples

D: FLK (*meaning* funny looking kid)
T: (leave blank; flag for alternative phrase)

See
coined terms
derogatory and inflammatory remarks
editing
risk management
slang

JCAHO

Abbreviation for *Joint Commission on Accreditation of Healthcare Organizations,* an independent, not-for-profit organization that develops organizational standards, awards accreditation decisions, and provides education and consultation to healthcare organizations. Previously known as Joint Commission on Accreditation of Hospitals (JCAH).

JD

Abbreviation for *Doctor of Jurisprudence* degree. No periods.

See degrees, academic

Jew

Use for both men and women; do not use *Jewess.* Adjective form: Jewish.

Jewett classification of bladder carcinoma

See cancer classifications

job descriptions

Do not confuse job descriptions with formal titles. Always lowercase job description names.

Debbie Vega is an administrative assistant at AAMT.

See titles

job titles

See titles

Johns Hopkins University
> *Johns* not *John* or *John's.*

Joint Commission on Accreditation of Healthcare Organizations
> *See* JCAHO

joule
> Pronounced *jewel.* SI unit of energy. Abbreviation: J (no period).
>
> *See* International System of Measuring Units

Jr., Jr
> *See* personal names, nicknames, and initials

July
> *See* months

June
> *See* months

junior
> Lowercase in references to academic class and member of class.
>
> She is a junior at Memorial High.
> The junior class dance is tomorrow night.

Jr., Jr
> *See* personal names, nicknames, and initials

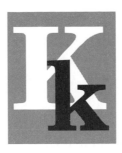

K

abbreviation for Kelvin
    See temperature, temperature scales

abbreviation for kilobyte
    Unit of measurement for a computer's memory capacity. One kilobyte is equal to 1024 bytes. Thus, 32K means 32 x 1024 bytes or 32,768, not 32,000. Do not space between the quantity and the abbreviation; do not use a period. Alternative abbreviation is *KB,* but *K* is preferred.

    64K *not* 64 K

chemical symbol for potassium
    See chemical nomenclature

    KCl (potassium chloride)

thousand
    Do not use *K* as an abbreviation for *thousand.*

    $30,000 *not* $30K
    platelets 340,000 *not* platelets 340K
    WBC 12,000 *not* WBC 12K

Karnofsky rating scale, Karnofsky status
    See scales

karyotype

See genetics terminology

KB

Abbreviation for *kilobyte* (unit of measurement for a computer's memory capacity), but *K* is preferred.

See K

Kelvin, kelvin

Capitalize when referring to the Kelvin temperature scale; lowercase when referring to a unit of temperature on that scale.

See
International System of Measuring Units
temperature, temperature scales

kilo-

Prefix meaning 1000 units of a measure. To convert to basic unit, move decimal point three places to the right, adding zeros as necessary.

11.8 kilograms = 11,800 grams

kilobyte

Abbreviation *K* is preferred to *KB*. Use abbreviated form with quantities.

kilocycle

Another term for *kilohertz*. Abbreviation: kc (no period).

kilogram

Metric term for 1000 grams (about 2.2 pounds or 35 ounces). Abbreviation: kg (no period). To convert to basic unit, move decimal point three places to the right, adding zeros as necessary. To convert to pounds, multiply by 2.2.

11.8 kg = 11,800 g
2 kg = 4.4 pounds

kilohertz
Metric term for 1000 hertz (1000 cycles per second); also known as *kilocycle*. Abbreviation: kHz (no period).

kilometer
Metric term for 1000 meters, approximately 3281 feet or 0.62 mile. Abbreviation: km (no period). To convert to basic unit, move decimal point three places to the right, adding zeros as necessary. To convert to miles, multiply by 0.62.

11.8 km = 11,800 m
4 km = 2.48 miles

kind, kinds
Use *that* with *kind, those* with *kinds*. Watch subject-verb agreement.

That kind of lab value is ambiguous.
Those kinds of decisions are difficult.

Kurtzke disability score
See scores

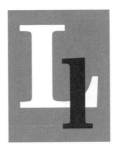

lab

Short form for *laboratory*. Acceptable if dictated, except in headings and subheadings.

laboratory data and values

Use numerals to express laboratory values.

Do not use commas to separate a lab value from the test it describes. When multiple lab results are given, separate related tests by commas, unrelated tests by periods (if uncertain, use periods). Use semicolons if entries in the series have internal commas.

White count 5.9, hemoglobin 14.6, hematocrit 43.1. Urine specific gravity 1.006, pH 6, negative dipstick.

Sodium 139, potassium 4.6, chloride 106, bicarb 28. White count 5.9, hemoglobin 14.6, hematocrit 43.1.

Blood work showed white count of 4800 with 58 segs, 7 bands, 24 lymphs, 8 monos, 2 eos, and 2 basos; hemoglobin 14.6 and hematocrit 43.1.

languages

Capitalize the proper names of languages and their dialects.

The patient speaks Laotian and English.
Her Cockney accent was difficult to understand.

laser

Acronym for *light amplification by stimulated emission of radiation,* which through widespread use has evolved into a word in its own right and thus is not capitalized.

last, latest

Use *latest* instead of *last* unless finality is intended.

The latest white count showed ...

Avoid *last* to indicate most recent month or day.

The patient was seen Thursday.
not The patient was seen last Thursday.

Latin abbreviations

drug-related abbreviations
See drug terminology

e.g., et al., etc., i.e., viz.
These Latin abbreviations are commonly used in English communications and need not be translated. Place a comma before and after the abbreviation (or its English equivalent).

e.g.	exempli gratia	for example
et al.	et alii	and others
etc.	et cetera	and so forth
i.e.	id est	that is
viz.	videlicet	that is, namely

She is fluent in several languages, e.g., French, Italian, and Spanish.
She is fluent in several languages, for example, French, Italian, and Spanish.

He continues to play football, basketball, baseball, tennis, etc., despite his knee injury.
He continues to play football, basketball, baseball, tennis, and so forth, despite his knee injury.

She continued to be uncooperative, i.e., she refused all treatment.
She continued to be uncooperative, that is, she refused all treatment.

He has numerous pets, viz., 8 dogs, 14 cats, 15 rabbits, 2 goats, and 3 llamas.
He has numerous pets, namely, 8 dogs, 14 cats, 15 rabbits, 2 goats, and 3 llamas.

See parenthetical expressions

Latino

Adjective referring to US citizen or resident of Latin-American or Spanish descent. *Hispanic* is also widely used, and *Mexican-American* may be preferred by those of Mexican descent.

See
Hispanic
Mexican-American
sociocultural designations

lay, lie

Do not confuse these terms.

lay

An action word meaning to place, to put, to deposit (something). It requires a direct object. Past tense and past participle *laid,* present participle *laying.* Note: *Lay* is also the past tense of *lie. See* lie *below.*

He laid the book on the table.

lie

Refers to a state of reclining. It does not take a direct object. Past tense *lay,* past participle *lain,* present participle *lying.*

She lay down for a rest.

le, la, l'

See personal names, nicknames, and initials

lead

verb
> Past tense is *led* not *lead*.

> She led the AMA's delegation to the White House.

cardiac leads
> Do not capitalize. *See* cardiology terminology

> lead aVF

length
> Express with numerals.

> The incision was 4 cm long.

> *See* numbers

lesbian, lesbianism
> Lowercase except in names of organizations.

less
> *See* fewer, less

less than (<)
> Use sign only in tables. Spell out the phrase in reports.

> She weighed less than 100 pounds.
> *not* She weighed <100 pounds.

letters

hyphens
> Use a hyphen to join some compound nouns with a number or single letter as a prefix; in other instances, separate them by a space. Check appropriate references for specific terms.

C-section
x-ray
R wave
T cell
Z line

When an unhyphenated word of this type acts as an adjective preceding a noun it becomes hyphenated.

T cell
but T-cell count

plurals
Use *'s* to form the plural of single letters.

p's and q's

See
compound modifiers
compound words

level
Position in a graded scale of values. Lowercase *level* and use arabic or roman numerals according to preference of system being referenced.

See scales

liability
See
professional liability insurance
risk management

lie
See lay, lie

like

preposition
In its prepositional form, *like* takes the objective case.

She looks like me.

conjunction
Use *like* to introduce a noun that is not followed by a verb. Use *as,* not *like,* to introduce a clause.

He exercises like an athlete.
He took the medication *as* he was instructed.
not He took the medication *like* he was instructed.

See as

line counts
A means by which transcription productivity may be measured; sometimes used as the basis for pay and/or charges.

Line lengths and type fonts vary from user to user, so meaningful usage requires specification of line length by converting to number of characters, i.e., 50-character line, 65-character line, 70-character line, etc.

Where line counts are used, AAMT prefers a 65-character line (based on AAMT's definition of a character).

There is no standard number of lines per minute of dictation.

AAMT discusses characters, words, lines, minutes of dictation, etc., in its press release titled, "AAMT Explores Quality and Quantity," which is reprinted in the text as Appendix F.

See
Appendix F, "AAMT Explores Quality and Quantity Issues"
Appendix R, "The Q-P Zone"
character
type font

line lengths
See line counts

Nothing is so fallacious as facts, except figures.
George Canning

line numbers
Lowercase line. Use ordinal or cardinal numbers.

line 12
12th line

linking verbs
See verbs

lists

run-on (horizontal) lists
Enclose arabic numbers in parentheses. Use commas or periods at the end of each, depending on usage or preference (note use of initial lower-cased or capital letter, depending on whether commas or periods separate entries).

Her past history includes (1) diabetes mellitus, (2) cholecystitis, (3) hiatal hernia.
or Her past history includes: (1) Diabetes mellitus. (2) Cholecystitis. (3) Hiatal hernia.

vertical (displayed) lists
Block style is preferred, with all entries aligned at left margin. If numbered, follow each arabic number by a period and then one character space; do not place numbers in parentheses. Capitalize the first letter of each entry whether or not numbered. Place a period at the end of each entry in the list.

1. Diabetes mellitus.
2. Cholecystitis.
3. Hiatal hernia.

FINAL DIAGNOSES
Adult-onset diabetes mellitus.
Gastroenteritis.

hanging indentation
Alternative form for displayed lists. Use arabic numerals and the following style:

1. Indent the first line of each item, and begin subsequent lines at the left margin.

2. This style works best with display lists that are presented in sentence form.

> *See*
> formats
> outlines
> series

liter
Basic unit of volume in metric system. One liter is equal to the volume occupied by one kilogram of water at 4 degrees Celsius. One liter is also equal to 1000 cubic centimeters, 1000 milliliters, 34 fluidounces, or 1.06 liquid quarts, 0.91 dry quart. Multiply by 1.06 to convert to liquid quarts. Multiply by 0.91 to convert to dry quarts. Multiply by 0.26 to convert to liquid gallons. Abbreviation: While either *L* or *l* is acceptable, *L* is preferred to *l* to avoid its being misread as the numeral *1* (one).

loci and locus symbols
See genetics terminology

> ***Words, like eyeglasses, blur everything***
> ***that they do not make clear.***
> Joseph Joubert

look-alikes
Terms that look like (and may or may not sound like) one another. Be alert so that you don't confuse such terms.

> affect   effect
> ileum   ilium

Read "Look-alikes and Soundalikes" column in *Journal of AAMT* for both an educational and humorous look at these phenomena.

See soundalikes

loupe magnification
See magnification

lowercase, lowercased
One word, no hyphen.

Ltd.
Term identifying a business entity as a limited company, i.e., one organized in a way that gives its owners limited liability.

See business names

-ly
Do not use a hyphen between adverbs that end in *-ly* and the adjectives they modify.

overly anxious parent

Do use a hyphen between adjectives that end in *-ly* and the adjectives they modify.

squirrelly-faced stuffed animal

See compound modifiers

lymphocyte and monoclonal antibody nomenclature
T lymphocytes (T cells) and B lymphocytes (B cells) are most common. *T* means thymus-derived, *B* means bursa-derived. In general, do not use extended forms.

hyphenation
Do not hyphenate except when used as adjectives preceding a noun.

T cells
T-cell count

pre- and pan-
Use a hyphen to join *pre* or *pan* to following letter or word.

pre-T cell
pan-B lymphocyte
pan-thymocyte

subsets of T lymphocytes
Use a virgule (not a hyphen) to express helper/inducer and cytotoxic/suppressor subsets of T lymphocytes.

helper/inducer T lymphocytes, a.k.a. helper cells, helper T lymphocytes
cytotoxic/suppressor T lymphocytes, a.k.a. suppressor cells

Use a hyphen (not a virgule or colon) in the phrase *helper-suppressor ratio.*

helper-suppressor ratio
not helper/suppressor ratio
not helper:suppressor ratio

surface antigens
Join on-line arabic numerals to the letter *T* to express surface antigens of T lymphocytes.

T3
T8
T11

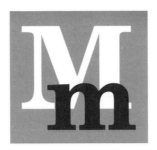

MA
　　Abbreviation for *Master of Arts* degree.

　　See degrees, academic

macro, macro-

macro
　　A keyboard command that incorporates two or more other commands or actions. Macros may be used to automate frequently performed tasks or to perform specialized calculations.

macro-
　　A prefix that is generally not hyphenated but joined directly to the term that follows. The usual exceptions apply.

　　macrobiotic
　　macrophage

　　See prefixes

magnification
　　Use a lowercased x and numerals in expressions of magnification. Space before and after the x.

　　x 20,000 magnification

loupe magnification
A loupe is a magnifying lens. *Loop* is **not** an acceptable alternative.

See International System of Measuring Units

mail
See USPS guidelines

main clause
Also known as *independent clause.*

See clauses

man, men
See age referents

March
See months

margins
See formats

master's degree
Lowercase this generic form, but use capitals when the specific form or abbreviation is used, e.g., Master of Arts (MA) degree or Master of Education (MEd) degree.

See degrees, academic

May
See months

MD
Abbreviation for *Doctor of Medicine*. Preferred style is without periods. If periods are used, do not space within the abbreviation (M.D., not M. D.). Set off the abbreviation by commas.

Thomas Gray, MD, of Modesto, California

mean, median
The *mean* is the average of a group of numbers. The *median* is the number at the midway point in a series of numbers listed in ascending or descending order.

Exam scores were 48, 49, 53, 88, and 92.
The mean score on the exam was 66.
The median score on the exam was 53.

measurements
See
International System of Measuring Units
numbers
units of measure

media
Plural of *medium,* so it takes a plural verb.

The contrast media were ...

median
See mean, median

Medicaid, Medicare
Federally funded programs for medical assistance. Capitalize initial letter only.

No one who has once taken the language under his care can ever again be really happy.
Thomas Lounsbury

medical language specialist
An alternative title for medical transcriptionist. Do not capitalize. Abbreviation: MLS (no periods).

See
Appendix O, "AAMT Model Job Description: Medical Transcriptionist"
medical transcriptionist
MLS

medical slang and jargon
See
jargon
slang

medical specialties
Do not capitalize the names of medical specialties or their variations that designate the practitioners of those specialties. These are common nouns, not proper nouns.

The orthopedist's evaluation ...
His specialty is cardiology.
The surgeon was Dr. Doolittle.

See nouns

A word after a word after a word is power.
Margaret Atwood

medical transcription

The process of interpreting and transcribing dictation by physicians and other healthcare professionals regarding patient assessment, work-up, therapeutic procedures, clinical course, diagnosis, prognosis, etc., into readable text, whether on paper or on computer, in order to document patient care and facilitate delivery of healthcare services. Abbreviation: MT (no periods).

See
Appendix L, "Medical Transcription as Communication"
Appendix M, "MTs: Partners in Medical Communication"
Appendix N, "The Myth of Medical Transcription"
Appendix O, "AAMT Model Job Description: Medical Transcriptionist"

The word is half his that speaks,
and half his that hears it.
Montaigne

medical transcriptionist

A medical language specialist who interprets and transcribes dictation by physicians and other healthcare professionals regarding patient assessment, workup, therapeutic procedures, clinical course, diagnosis, prognosis, etc., in order to document patient care and facilitate delivery of healthcare services. Abbreviation: MT (no periods).

AAMT's *Model Job Description: Medical Transcriptionist* gives additional information about the qualifications and responsibilities of medical transcriptionists.

Do not refer to a medical transcriptionist as a transcriber, which is a machine used by MTs for transcription purposes.

entry-level medical transcriptionist

There are a variety of interpretations and definitions for entry-level medical transcriptionist, depending on the work setting and the related type of transcription.

The Medical Transcriptionist Certification Program at AAMT adopted the following definition to describe an entry-level medical transcriptionist.

A medical language specialist who demonstrates that level of minimal competence which enables him/her to accurately interpret and transcribe routine patient care documentation by physicians and other healthcare professionals in a wide variety of work settings and specialty areas.

See
Appendix O, "AAMT Model Job Description: Medical Transcriptionist"
certified medical transcriptionist
medical language specialist
MT

medical transcriptionist certification
See Medical Transcriptionist Certification Program at AAMT

Medical Transcriptionist Certification Program at AAMT
Voluntary certification program administered by AAMT. Abbreviation: MTCP (no periods). It awards the CMT (certified medical transcriptionist) professional designation.

The mission of the MTCP is "to promote professional standards and improve the practice of medical transcription by giving special recognition to those professionals who demonstrate requisite knowledge, expertise, and performance through successful completion of the exam and who maintain certification through the fulfillment of stated requirements."

MTCP is responsible for setting the policies and standards and administering the certification and continuing education/recertification programs at AAMT. The Certification Commission has sole responsibility for certification and recertification standards, processes, eligibility, qualifications, and fees, as well as ultimate responsibility for exam content, scoring, and administration. The Examination Committee, which is responsible for developing, revising, and determining the final test items for the certification examination, reports to the Certification Commission.

For additional information on certification, contact the MTCP staff at AAMT: 800-982-2182, 209-551-0883, fax 209-551-9317.

See CMT

Medicare
See Medicaid, Medicare

medication dosages and doses
See drug terminology

medicolegal issues
See
audit trails
authentication
confidentiality
date dictated, date transcribed
dictated but not read
editing
Patient "Bill of Rights"
professional liability insurance
risk management
transcribed but not read

mega-
Prefix meaning 1 million units of a measure. Join without a hyphen. To convert to basic unit, move decimal point six places to the right, adding zeros as necessary.

3.8 megatons = 3,800,000 tons

men
See age referents

mEq
Abbreviation for *milliequivalent.* Use with numerals. Do not use periods. Do not add *s* for plural. Space between the numeral and the unit of measure.

20 mEq

meridians
Imaginary location lines that circle a globular structure, such as the eye, at right angles to its equator and touching both poles. Measured in units of 0 degrees to 180 degrees.

The eye was entered at the 160-degree meridian.

In acupuncture, meridians connect different anatomic sites.

meter

Basic unit of length in the metric system. Equal to 39.37 inches, usually rounded to 39.5 inches. To convert to inches, multiply by 39.37; to convert to yards, multiply by 1.1. Abbreviation: m (no period).

metric system

See
International System of Measuring Units
units of measure

Mexican-American

Adjective referring to US citizen or resident of Mexican descent.

See
Chicano
Hispanic
Latino
sociocultural designations

mg

Abbreviation for *milligram*. Do not use periods. Do not add *s* for plural. Space between the numeral and the abbreviation.

5 mg

micro-

Prefix meaning one-millionth of a unit. To convert to basic unit, move decimal point six places to the left.

14,596 mcg = 0.014596 g

This prefix is generally joined directly to the term that follows, i.e., it is not hyphenated. The usual exceptions apply.

micromanagement
microphage

See prefixes

mid, mid-

Mid can stand alone or serve as a prefix. When used as a prefix, it is usually connected to the word element without a hyphen, but there are the usual exceptions.

mid to lower lung fields
mid and distal palmar creases
midday
mid-Atlantic
mid-90s

See prefixes

middle initials

See personal names, nicknames, and initials

Mideast, Middle East

Capitalize as indicated. Adjective forms: Mideastern, Middle Eastern.

Midwest, Middle West

Capitalize as indicated. Adjective forms: Midwestern, Middle Western.

midnight

The end of a day, not the beginning of a new one. Do not capitalize. Do not use *12* with it.

Twin A was born at midnight, December 31, 1993; twin B at 12:14 a.m., January 1, 1994.

mile

Equal to 5280 feet or 1609 meters. Multiply by 1.6 to convert to kilometers. Do not abbreviate. Express with numerals.

14 miles = 22.4 km

miles per gallon (mpg)

Use abbreviation only when preceded by numerals. No periods; do not capitalize.

24 mpg

miles per hour (mph)

Use abbreviation only when preceded by numerals. No periods; do not capitalize.

84 mph

military terminology

military time
    See time

military titles
    See titles

military units

Use arabic ordinals and capitalize key words when expressed with figures.

The 2nd Infantry Division ...

milli-

Prefix meaning one-thousandth of a unit. To convert to basic unit, move decimal three places to the left.

1384 mg = 1.384 g

milliequivalent (mEq)

One-thousandth equivalent, i.e., the number of grams of a solute that are contained in one milliliter of a solution. Abbreviation: mEq (no periods; note capital *E*).

    20 mEq

milligram (mg)
    One-thousandth of a gram. Equals approximately 1/28,000 of an ounce. To convert to ounces, multiply by 0.000035. Abbreviation: mg (no period).

milliliter (ml)
    Unit of liquid measure. One-thousandth of a liter. Equal to approximately one-fifth of a teaspoon. To convert to teaspoons, multiply by 0.2. One fluidounce equals 30 ml. Abbreviation: ml (no period).

millimeter (mm)
    One-thousandth of a meter. Approximately 0.04 inch. To convert to inches, multiply by 0.04. One centimeter equals 10 mm. Abbreviation: mm (no period).

millisecond (ms or *msec)*
    One thousandth of a second. Abbreviation: ms *or* msec (no periods).

minus, minus sign (-)
    Express with a hyphen, not a dash; do not space between the hyphen and numeral.

    -40 *not* —40 *not* - 40

    Write out *minus* if you are not certain the symbol will be noticeable or clear.

    minus 40

    Write out *minus* to indicate below-zero temperatures.

    minus 38 degrees *not* -38 degrees

plus/minus
    Express as *plus or minus* or *plus/minus,* not +/- except in tables.

    See negative sign

Miss
Plural: Misses.

See titles

missing antecedents
See pronouns

ml
Abbreviation for *milliliter.* Use with numerals. Do not use periods. Do not add *s* for plural. Space between the numeral and the unit of measure.

50 ml

MLS
Abbreviation for *medical language specialist.* No periods.

It is not appropriate to use *MLS* following a name because doing so gives it the appearance of being a recognized professional credential, which it is not. The only recognized professional credential for medical transcriptionists (and therefore for medical language specialists) is CMT (certified medical transcriptionist).

Rhonda Williams, medical language specialist
not Rhonda Williams, MLS

See
CMT
credentials, professional
medical language specialist

mm
Abbreviation for *millimeter,* unit of measure for length, breadth, width, depth, height, etc. Use with numerals. Do not use periods. Do not add *s* for plural. Space between the numeral and the unit of measure.

50 mm

mmHg, mm Hg

Abbreviation for *millimeters of mercury*. Use with pressure readings (blood pressure, tourniquet pressure, etc.). If the phrase is not dictated, use of the abbreviation is optional. Note there are no periods, and you may space or not between *mm* and *Hg* (be consistent). AAMT prefers the non-spaced form.

D: BP 110/90
T: BP 110/90 mmHg
or BP 110/90

model job descriptions

medical transcriptionist

The *AAMT Model Job Description: Medical Transcriptionist* is designed to assist human resource managers, department managers, supervisors, and others in recruiting, supervising, and evaluating individuals in medical transcription positions. It provides a practical compilation of the basic job responsibilities of a medical transcriptionist.

supervisor of medical transcription

The development of a model job description for medical transcription supervisors is in process by AAMT. Contact AAMT for further information.

See Appendix O, "AAMT Model Job Description: Medical Transcriptionist"

model numbers

See equipment terms

modifiers

See
adjectives
adverbs
compound modifiers
eponyms
prefixes
suffixes

molarity
See solutions

Monday
See days of the week

> ## When I get a little money, I buy books;
> ## and if any is left, I buy food and clothes.
> Desiderius Erasmus

money
Express exact amounts of dollars and cents with numerals, using a decimal point to separate dollars and cents. When written out, lowercase all terms.

$4.56
four dollars and fifty-six cents

amounts less than $1
Use numerals; spell out and lowercase *cents*. Do not use decimal form. Do not use dollar sign ($). Do not use cent sign (¢) except in tabular matter.

8 cents *not* $.08 *not* 8¢
20 cents *not* $.20 *not* 20¢

in tables: 20¢ *not* .20¢ *not* $.20

amounts over $1
Use dollar sign ($) preceding the dollar amount, and separate dollars and cents by a decimal point. Do not use a decimal following the dollar amount if cents are not included.

$1.08
$1.20
$40

verb-subject agreement
Money expressions take a singular verb when they are thought of as a sum, a plural verb when they are thought of as individual bills and coins.

A million dollars is a lot of money.
The 50 quarters were stacked on the dresser.

possessive adjectives
Use *'s* or *s'*, whichever is appropriate, with units of money used as possessive adjectives. Do not use possessive form with compound adjectives.

one dollar's worth
two cents' worth
two-dollar bill

ranges
Repeat the dollar sign or cent sign but do not repeat the word forms. Use *to* instead of a hyphen with dollar-sign or cent-sign forms. Use *to* with word forms.

$4 to $5 *not* $4-$5
10¢ to 15¢ *not* 10¢-15¢
4 to 5 dollars *not* 4-5 dollars
10 to 15 cents *not* 10-15 cents

monoclonal antibody nomenclature
See lymphocyte and monoclonal antibody nomenclature

months
Capitalize the names of months. Do not abbreviate except in tables and in military style, and even then, do not abbreviate March, April, May, June, July, unless all of the months are expressed as three-letter abbreviations without ending periods.

month	*tabular abbreviation*
January	Jan. *or* Jan
February	Feb. *or* Feb
March	March *or* Mar
April	April *or* Apr
May	May *or* May

June	June *or* Jun
July	July *or* Jul
August	Aug. *or* Aug
September	Sept. *or* Sep
October	Oct. *or* Oct
November	Nov. *or* Nov
December	Dec. *or* Dec

See dates

more than (>)

Use the sign only in tables. Spell out the phrase in reports.

She weighed more than 300 pounds.
not She weighed >300 pounds.

Mount

Abbreviate or spell out in proper names according to common or preferred usage related to entity in question. Of course, spell out and lowercase generic uses.

Mount Vernon
Mt. Shasta

mpg

Abbreviation for *miles per gallon.* Do not use periods. Do not add *s* for plural. Space between the numeral and the abbreviation.

40 mpg

mph

Abbreviation for *miles per hour.* Do not use periods. Do not add *s* for plural. Space between the numeral and the abbreviation.

40 mph

Mr., Mr
Abbreviation for *Mister.* Courtesy title for a man. It may be expressed with or without the ending period. Plural: Messrs.

See titles

Mrs., Mrs
Courtesy title for a married or widowed woman. May be written without the ending period. Plural: Mmes.

See titles

ms, msec
See msec, ms

Ms., Ms
Courtesy title for a woman or girl. May be written without the ending period. No plural; repeat *Ms.* before each name.

Ms. Blakeman, Ms. Olaes, and Ms. White are clerical assistants at AAMT.

See titles

MS
Abbreviation for *Master of Science* degree.

See degrees, academic

msec, ms
Abbreviations for *millisecond.* Do not use periods. Do not add *s* for plural. Space between the numeral and the abbreviation.

150 ms
280 msec

MT

Abbreviation for *medical transcription* and for *medical transcriptionist* (also for medical technologist, music therapist, massage therapist). No periods. Plural: MTs. Possessive: MT's (singular) or MTs' (plural).

It is not appropriate to use *MT* following a name because doing so gives it the appearance of being a recognized professional credential, which it is not. The only recognized professional credential for medical transcriptionists is CMT (certified medical transcriptionist).

Rhonda Williams, medical transcriptionist
not Rhonda Williams, MT

See
CMT
credentials, professional
medical transcriptionist

MT Reference Library

See references

MTCP

See Medical Transcriptionist Certification Program at AAMT

mucus, mucous

Mucus is the noun form; *mucous,* the adjective form.

She coughed up mucus.
The mucous discharge is of concern.
Mucus-type tissue was noted. (Use noun form with *-type.*)
The wound is mucus-producing. (*Mucus* is object of present
    participle verb, so noun form, not adjective form, must be used.)

multiplication symbol

See x

murmurs, murmur grades

See cardiology terminology

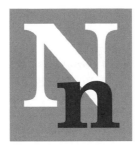

namely

Latin equivalent is *viz.*

See Latin abbreviations

names

brand name

Nonlegal term for *trademark*. Capitalize brand names. *See* trademark *below*.

Adaptic gauze dressing

generic name

Established, nonproprietary name for a drug, suture, instrument, etc. Its use is unrestricted. Do not capitalize generic names; they are common nouns.

catgut sutures
aspirin
milk of magnesia
imipramine

proper name

Specific name of a person, place, or thing. Capitalize most proper names. (Occasional exceptions, e.g., e.e. cummings, exist.)

the White House

Do not use an apostrophe in plural forms of proper names.

The Smiths were referred by …
All Toms, Dicks, and Marys were there.

trade name
Broader term than *trademark*. Identifies manufacturer, but not necessarily the product or process. Capitalize trade names, but do not use all capitals even if the manufacturer does.

Bayer aspirin
Dr. Scholl's foot powder

> ### *If names are not correct, language will not be in accordance with the truth of things.*
> Confucius

trademark
Manufacturer's name for a product or process that it has patented and protected by law against use by competitor. Also known as *brand name* or *proprietary name.*

Capitalize the initial letter of the trademark or brand name of drugs, sutures, instruments, etc. In the case of oddities such as pHisoHex, where there is eccentric use of capitals, it is acceptable either (1) to match the manufacturer's presentation or (2) to use initial capital only. However, when the manufacturer uses all capitals, use an initial capital only so as not to give undue attention to the term in a medical report. It is not necessary to use the trademark symbols (™ or ®).

Vicryl
pHisoHex *or* Phisohex
RhoGAM *or* Rhogam
Ligaclip (*not* LIGACLIP [the manufacturer's style])

Do not capitalize adjectives and common nouns associated with trademark or brand names.

Adaptic gauze dressing
Tylenol tablets

intravenous Valium
running Dacron sutures

nomenclatures

Numerous nomenclatures, or naming systems, are used in medicine to promote the consistent, correct, and stable naming of entities; only selected ones are addressed in this style book.

AAMT guidelines for expressing nomenclatures in transcription take into account recommendations and guidelines from reliable sources, e.g., *AMA Manual of Style* and the American Diabetes Association, as well as equipment capabilities and deficiencies (for example, in relation to subscripts and superscripts) in order to promote consistency, ease of use, and communication. Thus, official forms, as well as forms within manuscripts, may differ.

See specific entries, including
building, structure, and room names
business names
cancer classifications
cardiology terminology
chemical nomenclature
classifications
clotting factor terms
diabetes mellitus terminology
disease names
drug terminology
electroencephalographic terms
eponyms
equipment terms
family relationship names
genetics terminology
genus and species names
geographic names
hepatitis nomenclature
hormones
International System of Measuring Units
lymphocyte and monoclonal antibody nomenclature
medical specialties
north, south, east, west
nouns
obstetrics terminology
personal names, nicknames, and initials
plant names

pulmonary and respiratory terms
scales
scores
Spanish names
titles
units of measure
virus names

nano-
Prefix meaning one-billionth of a unit. To convert to basic unit, move decimal point nine places to the left.

4987870984.4 nanoseconds = 4.9878709844 seconds

nation, national
Lowercase except when part of a proper name or formal title.

The nation's capital is Washington, DC.
National Medical Transcriptionist Week
Face the Nation

national productivity standard
See productivity

nationalities
Capitalize proper names of nationalities, peoples, races, tribes, etc. Use hyphenation according to preferred usage (check appropriate references).

American
British
Canadian
French Canadian

Do not use derogatory or inflammatory terms associated with nationalities except in direct quotes that are essential to the report. Bring inappropriate usage to attention of those responsible for risk management.

See sociocultural designations

negative findings

Negative findings are those within normal limits; they are also referred to as normal findings. Positive findings are those not within normal limits.

Transcribe all findings, whether identified as negative, normal, or positive. Do not exclude normal or negative findings when they are dictated. Negative or normal findings may be as important to diagnosis and treatment as are positive or abnormal findings. Recording such findings provides medicolegal documentation that the related tests or exams were done and reduces the unnecessary repetition of tests or procedures to determine findings, in turn reducing healthcare costs.

See positive findings

negative sign (-)

Do not use except in tables or special applications, e.g., blood nomenclature.

blood type O-

See minus, minus sign

neither...nor, either...or

See either...or, neither...nor

neonate, newborn

See age referents

New York Heart Association classification of cardiac failure

See cardiology terminology

nicknames

See personal names, nicknames, and initials

nineteen-hundreds
Preferred form is *1900s.*

See years, decades, centuries

no one, none

no one
Takes a singular verb.

No one expects him to recover full use of the arm.

none
May be singular (*not one, no one, no single one*) or plural (*no two, no amount, not any*), taking singular or plural verbs and pronouns as the case may be.

We tried to identify the bleeding site; none was found.
We found four bleeding sites; none were cauterized.

Use context to determine if singular or plural form is intended. If either could be used, assume it is singular and use singular verbs and pronouns.

In the phrase *none of,* the object of the preposition *of* determines whether construction is singular or plural.

None of *the findings are* conclusive.
None of *it makes* sense.

No.,
Abbreviation and symbol for *number.* Note that the abbreviation capitalizes the initial letter and has an ending period.

position or rank
Use the abbreviation or symbol with a figure to indicate position or rank.

He is No. 4 on the appointment list.
or He is #4 on the appointment list.

model and serial numbers
Use the symbol with arabic numerals.

model #8546
serial #185043

street addresses
Do not use the abbreviation or symbol before the number in street addresses.

166 Wallingford Avenue
not No. 166 Wallingford Avenue
not #166 Wallingford Avenue

suites, apartments, rooms
Use the abbreviation or symbol in suite, apartment, room, or similar number designations, when the noun designation is not used.

#104 *or* No. 104 *or* Apt. 104 *not* Apt. #104

schools, fire companies, lodges
Do not use the abbreviation or symbol in names of schools, fire companies, lodges, or similar numbered units.

Public School 4
Engine 3

sizes of instruments or sutures
Do not use the abbreviation or symbol if "number" is not dictated. Either is optional (with the symbol preferred to the abbreviation) if "number" is dictated. Be consistent.

5-French catheter, #5-French catheter, No. 5-French catheter
3-0 Vicryl, #3-0 Vicryl, No. 3-0 Vicryl

See numbers

nomenclatures
See names

none
> *See* no one, none

nonmetric units of measure
> *See* units of measure

noon
> The middle of the day. Lowercase. Do not use *12* in conjunction with it.
>
> The infant was born at noon, January 14, 1994.

normal findings
> Also referred to as *negative findings*.
>
> *See*
> negative findings
> positive findings

north, northern, North, Northern
> *See* north, south, east, west

north, south, east, west (and their variations)

compass points and directions
> Lowercase the term when referring to compass points or directions.
>
> Their house faces south.
> They headed east from California.
> They proceeded in a northerly direction.

geographic regions
> Capitalize the term when it is part of a proper name of a state, country, region, or location.
>
> South Korea
> East Germany
> South Carolina

South Pole
Northern Hemisphere

Capitalize the term when referring to US coastal regions, but lower-case it when referring to the shoreline itself. (Use *the Coast* for references to the West Coast only.)

He is from the East Coast.
Some areas of the east coast have had severe storm damage.
She returned to the Coast by air, landing in Los Angeles.

Capitalize the term when referring to geographic regions of the United States or when referring to a widely recognized region within a state, but lowercase it when referring to a less commonly recognized region within a state.

She is from the Southwest.
She is from Northern California.
He is from northern New Hampshire.
He is from the Midwest but has lived in the East for 20 years.
She exaggerates her Southern accent.

Capitalize the term when referring to a native or resident of a geographic region of the United States.

The AAMT staff are a bunch of Westerners.

Capitalize the term when it is part of a phrase that is commonly used in reference to a city's section, but lowercase it if it is not a common designation.

She grew up on Chicago's South Side.
He lives on the south side of town.

Capitalize *Northwest* in reference to that territorial section of Canada.

Northwest Territories

Capitalize *West / Western* when referring to the Occident, *East / Eastern* when referring to the Orient.

Western dress is increasingly common in Eastern countries.

ideological divisions
Capitalize *East/Eastern* and *West/Western* when referring to ideological divisions of the world.

He was born in what was then an Eastern bloc country.

time zones
Most references capitalize *Eastern* when used in reference to a time zone, but some do not. Be consistent.

Eastern time zone *or* eastern time zone
Eastern daylight time *or* eastern daylight time

See
geographic names
time zones

not only...but also
Correlative conjunctions. Check usage for parallelism; recast as necessary. If *also* is omitted, insert it or some other word(s) for balance.

D: He could not only be stubborn but offensive.
T: He could be not only stubborn but also offensive.
or He could be not only stubborn but offensive as well.

nouns
Abbreviation *n* is used in this book where it is necessary to identify noun forms.

mucus (n)
mucous (adj)

Proper nouns name specific persons, places, and things. All other nouns are common nouns. It may help to think of proper nouns as brand names and common nouns as generic terms. Do not capitalize common nouns in an effort to give them the stature of proper nouns.

He was admitted to *St. Mary's Hospital.* (proper noun)
She was seen in the *emergency room* (common noun) of St. Mary's Hospital.

Nouns usually are subjects or objects of a sentence. Sometimes, they may be modifiers.

She became ill while attending AAMT's *educators* conference. (*not* educators' conference)

Use the possessive form for a noun or pronoun that precedes a gerund (verb ending in *-ing* and used as a noun).

His dieting is a problem.
The *patient's screaming* disturbed other patients.

Use the possessive form for a noun involving time or money that is used as a possessive adjective.

The pain was of three months' duration.

collective noun
Represents a collection of persons or things regarded as a unit. Usage determines whether the collective noun is singular or plural. It is singular and takes a singular verb when the total group it represents is emphasized. It is plural and takes a plural verb when the individuals making up the group are emphasized.

examples of collective nouns
board (of directors)
class
committee
couple
family
group
majority
number
pair
set
staff
team

The group is meeting frequently throughout its stay.
The group of patients were female. *(each was female)*

A number of adhesions were present. *(individual adhesions were present, not a collective adhesion)*
The number of adhesions was minimal.

The couple were injured in a plane crash.
but The couple has an appointment with the geneticist.

Treat units of measure as singular collective nouns that take singular verbs.

Twenty milliequivalents of KCl was given.

See
compound modifiers
compound words
names
plurals
verb-subject agreement

noun-verb agreement
See verb-subject agreement

November
See months

n.p.o.
See drug terminology

n.r.
See drug terminology

numbers
Express numbers as numerals (arabic or roman) or words, according to rules of style. A numeral is a symbol representing a number.

The number *four* is represented by the numeral *4*.

cardinal numbers

Numbers used to indicate quantity. Use arabic numerals to express quantities accompanied by a unit of measure, to express ages and other vital statistics, to express lab values, and in any other instance when it is important to communicate quickly and clearly the number referenced. For uses not covered (explicitly or implicitly) by guidelines stated in this entry or in cross-references, spell out whole numbers *one* through *nine,* use figures for 10 and above.

> 5 inches
> 4-year-old patient
> pH 6
> respirations 16

> She has four cats although she is allergic to them.
> We removed 11 lymph nodes.

ordinal numbers

Numbers used to indicate position in a series or order. Spell out *first* through *ninth* when they indicate sequence in time or location. Starting with *10th,* use figures. Use *1st, 2nd, 3rd, 4th,* etc., when used as part of a series: 4th cranial nerve, 7th Fleet, 1st Sgt. Do not use a period with ordinal numbers.

> The fifth specimen was ...
> She was in her ninth month of pregnancy.
> His return visits are scheduled for the 15th and 25th of next month.
> The 4th cranial nerve ...

arabic numerals

Also *Arabic.* Arabic numerals include 0, 1, 2, 3, 4, 5, 6, 7, 8, 9. *See* cardinal numbers *above.*

Most numerals used in medicine are expressed as arabic numerals. Therefore, a general rule is to use arabic numerals unless roman are specified. *See* roman numerals *below, as well as specific entries and appropriate references.*

adjacent numerals

When a quantitative number precedes a number accompanying a unit of measure, write out the quantity and use numerals with the unit of measure.

two 8-inch drains
six 2-gauge needles

Use a comma to separate adjacent unrelated numerals if neither can be readily expressed in words and the sentence cannot be readily reworded.

In March 1991, 1038 patients were seen in the emergency room.

at beginning of sentence
Do not use a numeral at the beginning of a sentence. Spell out the number, or recast the sentence to place the numeral elsewhere.

D: 11 of her children are living.
T: Eleven of her children are living.

at end of line
Do not separate numerals from the terms they accompany, so do not allow a numeral to end one line and its accompanying term to begin the next.

..................................grade 2.
not
..................................grade
2.

multiple digits
Use a comma to separate groups of three numerals in numbers of 5 digits or more, but omit the commas if decimals are used. Omit the comma in 4-digit numerals.

Platelet count was 354,000.
White count was 7100.
12345.67

When dictated in a form such as "four point two thousand" or "five point eight million," numerals may be transcribed in one of two ways:

4.2 thousand
or 4200

5.8 million
or 5,800,000

hyphens
Use hyphens in compound numbers from 21 to 99 when they are written out.

thirty-four
one hundred fifty-three

Use a hyphen when numbers are used with words as a compound modifier preceding a noun.

5-cm incision
two-week history
13-year-old female

Use a hyphen to join some compound nouns with a number as a prefix. Check appropriate references for specific terms.

3-D images

plurals
Use *'s* to form the plural of single-digit numerals. Add *s* without an apostrophe to form the plural of multiple-digit numbers, including years.

4 x 4's
She is in her 20s.
She was born in the 1940s.

proper names
Use words or figures for numbers in proper names, according to the entity's preference.

20th Century Insurance
Three Dollar Cafe

series
Use numerals if the information is significant. Even with nonsignificant information, use numerals if at least one of them is more than nine or is a mixed or decimal fraction.

She has 4 cats, 2 dogs, and 18 hamsters.

spelled out
Spell out numbers that begin a sentence, or recast the sentence.

Forty milliequivalents of KCl was given.
or KCl 40 mEq was given.
not 40 mEq of KCl was given.

The 20th Century Insurance company ...
not 20th Century Insurance ...

Spell out casual (nonspecific) numeric expressions.

She described hundreds of symptoms.

Do not place commas between words expressing a number.

four hundred forty-eight
not four hundred, forty-eight

roman numerals
    Also *Roman.* Do not use periods with roman numerals. Seven letters make up the roman numeral system. Capital letters are used except in special circumstances, e.g., lowercased letters (i, v, x, etc.) are used for page numbers for preliminary material (contents pages, preface, etc.) in a book.

    I = 1
    V = 5
    X = 10
    L = 50
    C = 100
    D = 500
    M = 1000

    When a letter follows a letter of greater value, it increases the value of the preceding letter.

    VI (5 + 1 = 6)

    When a letter precedes a letter of greater value it diminishes the value of the following letter.

    IV (5 - 1 = 4)

A bar over a letter indicates multiplication by 1000.

$\overline{X}$ = 10,000

Following are some common applications that use roman numerals. To determine arabic or roman numeral usage for other topics, check the arabic section of this topic, as well as other appropriate entries or references.

cranial nerves: Roman numerals remain preferred in cranial nerve designations, but arabic numerals may be used.

cranial nerves I-XII
cranial nerves 1-12

eponyms: Roman numerals are generally used with eponyms, but check references for guidance with specific terms. Do not place a hyphen between the eponym and the numeral.

She had a LeFort I maxillary reconstruction.

operations: Roman numerals are used in some operation names.

Billroth II anastomosis

types: Roman numerals are used in certain designations.

type II diabetes mellitus

wars, people, animals: Roman numerals are used for wars, people and animals.

World War II
Henry Ford III
Rover II

See specific entries, including:
addresses
ages
cancer classifications
cardiology terminology
classifications
dates

decimals, decimal units
drug terminology
fractions
International System of Measuring Units
laboratory data and values
lists
No., #
outlines
page numbers
percent
proportions
range
ratio
scales
scores
Social Security number
street names and numbers
telephone numbers
temperature, temperature scales
units of measure
USPS guidelines
vertebra
years, decades, centuries

number of

A collective noun that may be singular or plural. If preceded by *the,* it takes a singular verb. If preceded by *a,* it takes a plural verb.

The number of adhesions was minimal.
A number of adhesions were present.

number sign/symbol/abbreviation (#, No.)

See No., #

numerals

See numbers, *as well as specific topics for specific uses*

NYHA classification of cardiac failure

See cardiology terminology

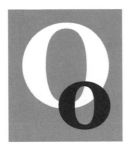

obscenities, profanities, vulgarities

Avoid except as part of direct quotations that are essential to the report. Bring them to attention of risk manager.

See
editing
risk management

The thoughtless are rarely wordless.
Howard W. Newton

obstetrics terminology

abort, abortion

The *AMA Manual of Style* prefers the term *terminate* to *abort,* but AAMT does not recommend making this editorial change if *abort* is dictated.

D: abort
T: abort (*not* terminate)

cesarean section

Not *Cesarean, caesarean,* or *Caesarean.* Brief form is *C-section,* but do not use it unless it is dictated, and even then do not use it in operative title section of operative reports or discharge summaries.

fundal height
Distance from symphysis pubis to dome (top) of uterus. Expressed in centimeters. After 12th week of pregnancy, the number should equal the number of weeks of pregnancy, but it may indicate large-for-date fetus or multiple fetuses.

Fundal height is 28 cm.

GPA terminology
GPA is abbreviation for *gravida, para, aborta.* Accompanied by arabic numbers, *G, P,* and *A* (or *Ab*) describe the patient's obstetric history. Roman numerals are not appropriate.

G	gravida (number of pregnancies)	
P	para (number of births of viable offspring)	
A *or* Ab	aborta (abortions)	

nulligravida	gravida 0	no pregnancies
primigravida	gravida 1, G1	1 pregnancy
secundigravida	gravida 2, G2	2 pregnancies
nullipara	para 0	no deliveries of viable offspring

Separate GPA sections by commas. Alternatively, spell out the terms, using lowercase.

Obstetric history: G4, P3, A1.
or Obstetric history: gravida 4, para 3, aborta 1.

When one or more of the numbers is 0, the preferred form is to write out the terms.

gravida 2, para 0, aborta 2

station
Term designating the location of the presenting fetal part in the birth canal. Expressed as -5 to +5, representing the number of centimeters below or above an imaginary plane through the ischial spine (station 0 is at the plane).

TPAL terminology
System used to describe obstetrics history of a patient.

T   term infants
P   premature infants
A   abortions
L   living children

Separate TPAL numbers by hyphens.

Obstetric history: 4-2-2-4.

Alternatively, spell out the terms, as follows:

Obstetric history: 4 term infants, 2 premature infants, 2 abortions, 4 living children.

Sometimes, GPA terminology is combined with TPAL terminology.

The patient is gravida 3, 3-0-0-3.

occupational titles
See titles

ocean
Capitalize only when a part of a proper name. Lowercase other uses.

Pacific Ocean
Arctic Ocean
He became ill while on an ocean cruise.
The Pacific and Atlantic oceans ...

o'clock
See
a.m., AM; p.m., PM
clock referents
time

October
See months

o.d., OD

o.d.
> *See* drug terminology

OD
> Abbreviation for *oculus dexter,* meaning *right eye,* and for *Doctor of Optometry* degree. In either usage, capitalize and do not use periods.

> *See* degrees, academic

off
> Preposition. Do not follow by *of.*

> He fell off the roof.
> *not* He fell off of the roof.

oh
> Do not capitalize except at beginning of sentence. Do not use *O* instead.

oncogenes
> *See* genetics terminology

one another
> *See* each other, one another

only
> Take care to place *only* next to the word it is modifying, or its meaning may be confused. Its misplacement makes it a squinting modifier.

> D: He only walked two blocks.
> T: He walked only two blocks.

> *See* adverbs

operate, operate on

A surgeon operates **on** a patient, and a patient is operated **on**. Add *on* even if not dictated.

D: The patient was operated without incident.
T: The patient was operated on without incident.

operative report

One of the basic 4 reports. Abbreviation: op (no period).
Typical content headings in an operative report include:

preoperative diagnosis
postoperative diagnosis
reason for operation
operation performed
surgeon
assistants
anesthesiologist
anesthesia
indications for procedure
findings
procedure
complications
specimens
estimated blood loss
instrument and sponge counts

See
Appendix A, "Sample Reports"
basic 4 reports
formats

***The epithet* beautiful *is used by surgeons
to describe an operation which
their patients describe as ghastly.***
George Bernard Shaw

oral

In reference to language, *oral* refers only to words that are spoken. *Verbal* refers to words used in any manner, e.g., spoken, written, typed, printed, signed.

ordinal numbers

See numbers

organizations

See business names

originator

One who "speaks" the document to be transcribed, whether it be a report, letter, manuscript, or other. Also called *dictator* or *author.*

OS

Abbreviation for *oculus sinister,* left eye. Capitalize; do not use periods.

ounce

Equal to 28 grams. To convert to grams, multiply by 28.

2 ounces = 56 grams

Write out; do not use abbreviation (*oz.*) except in tables. Express accompanying numbers as numerals. Do not use a comma or other punctuation between units for pounds and units for ounces.

The infant weighed 13 pounds 2 ounces

fluidounce, fluid ounce

Apothecary ounce (used in USP) equals 8 dr., 31.10349 g, 2 table-spoons, 6 teaspoons. Avoirdupois ounce equals 28.35 g. Metric equivalent is approximately 30 ml, so to convert to milliliters, multiply by 30.

4 fluidounces = 120 ml

See
grain
gram

Outerbridge scale
    See scales

outlines
    Use for displayed (vertical) lists with two or more values and levels, alternating numerals and letters. Each level should have two or more entries. Use a period after divisional numerals and letters that are not in parentheses; do not use periods following numerals and letters that are in parentheses.

two-level outline

        1.
            a.
            b.
        2.

    or

        I.
            A.
            B.
        II.

three-level outline

        1.
            a.
            b.
                (1)
                (2)
        2.

    or

I.
    A.
    B.
        1.
        2.
II.

four-level outline

I.
    A.
    B.
        1.
        2.
            a.
            b.
II.

more than four levels

Repeat sublevels, placing numerals and letters in parentheses, e.g., a six-level outline:

I.
    A.
    B.
        1.
        2.
            a.
            b.
                (1)
                (2)
                    (a)
                    (b)

II.

See
formats
lists
series

over

When *over* means *more than,* replace it with same.

D: She reports over five operations but is unclear about the precise number.
T: She reports more than five operations but is unclear about the precise number.

When *over* may mean *more than* or *for a period of* and you can determine the intended meaning, replace *over* with the more precise term.

D: The rash persisted over two weeks.
T: The rash persisted for over two weeks.
or The rash persisted over a two-week period.

If you cannot determine the meaning, transcribe as dictated.

The rash persisted over two weeks.

Use a virgule to express *over* in expressions such as the following.

D: blood pressure 160 over 100
T: blood pressure 160/100

D: grade 1 over 4 murmur
T: grade 1/4 murmur

See
prefixes
prepositions

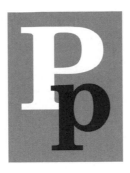

pacemaker codes
> *See* cardiology terminology

pack-year history of smoking
> Smoking history expressed as amount equal to packs smoked per day times number of years smoking. Use numerals and hyphens as follows:

> 20-pack-year history

> In above example, patient's smoking history is equivalent to 1 pack per day for 20 years or 2 packs per day for 10 years or 5 packs per day for 4 years, etc.

> ### *I never smoked a cigarette until I was nine.*
> H.L. Mencken

page numbers
> Lowercase *page* and use arabic numerals.

> His history is detailed on page 2 of the report dated January 4, 1994.

> Lowercased roman numerals (i, v, x, etc.) refer to page numbers for preliminary material (contents pages, preface, etc.) in a book.

Pap test, Pap smear

Pap is brief form for *Papanicolaou* and may be used if dictated. If full word is dictated, transcribe in full.

Papanicolaou test, Papanicolaou smear

See Pap test, Pap smear

para

See obstetrics terminology

paragraphs

See formats

parallel construction

Elements of a series should be parallel, e.g., nouns with nouns, gerunds with gerunds. Edit appropriately.

D: Hobbies include knitting, sewing, and she likes to ride horses.
T: Hobbies include knitting, sewing, and riding horses.

With correlative conjunctions (either...or, neither...nor, not only... but also, both...and), use parallel construction on each side of the coordinating conjunction.

D: She has both pain and she has fever.
T: She has both pain and fever.

unparallel series

Also known as bastard enumeration.

See series

parentheses ()

Parentheses are used to provide parenthetical (incidental or supplementary) information that is not closely related to the rest of the sentence. They may or may not be dictated.

Use parentheses sparingly. If the parenthetical information is closely related to the rest of the sentence, use commas instead.

A great deal of swelling was present, more so on the left than the right.

not A great deal of swelling was present (more so on the left than the right).

brackets ([])
Use brackets around a parenthetical insertion that contains a parenthetical insertion. Follow the rules for parentheses. *See* braces *below*.

The chemical formula for chlorphenoxamine hydrochloride is 2-[1-(4-chlorophenyl)-1-phenylethoxy]-*N*,*N*-dimethylethanamine hydrochloride.

braces ({})
Use braces around a parenthetical insertion that contains both a bracketed and a parenthetical insertion. Follow the rules for parentheses. *See* brackets *above*.

The chemical formula for hydroxychloroquine sulfate is 7-chloro-4-{4-[ethyl(2-hydroxyethyl)amino]-1-methylbutylamino}-quinoline sulfate.

capitalization
If the parenthetical entry is within a sentence, begin it with a lowercased letter and omit closing punctuation whether or not it is a complete sentence.

Further past history shows outpatient pulmonary function tests with a forced vital capacity of 2.57 liters (that is equal to 62% of predicted) and an FEV of 0.98 liters.

A parenthetical entry that stands on its own (is not within a sentence) must be a complete sentence; start it with a capital letter and end it with closing punctuation inside the closing parenthesis.

Pelvic ultrasound was read as intrauterine changes consistent with pyometra. (It is difficult to believe that this diagnosis could be made on the basis of an ultrasound.)

comma
Do not precede a parenthesis mark by a comma. If a comma is required following the parenthetical information, it must be placed after the closing parenthesis mark.

The patient is improving (despite her repeated insistence that she is dying), and we plan to discharge her to an extended care facility next week.

enumerated items within a sentence
Use arabic numerals within parentheses to enumerate items within a sentence. Separate the enumerated entries by commas or semicolons.

He has a long history of known diagnoses, including (1) chronic silicosis, (2) status post left thoracotomy, (3) arteriosclerotic cardiovascular disease.

singular or plural forms
Sometimes parentheses are used around the letter(s) *s* or *es* to indicate that the noun can be either singular or plural. When the noun is the subject, it takes a singular verb since the *s* or *es* is parenthetical. Sometimes the awkwardness of this construction can be avoided by using just the plural noun.

The parenthetical letter(s) indicates the noun is either singular or plural. *(letter...indicates)*
or The parenthetical letters indicate the noun is either singular or plural. *(letters...indicate)*

See
parenthetical expressions
periods
question marks
series

parenthetical expressions
Expressions that interrupt the flow of the sentence. They are set off by commas (not parentheses, as one would expect by their name). Even the commas may be omitted if their absence will not confuse the reader.

A great deal of swelling was present, *more so on the left than on the right.*
Ultimately this cleared, *however,* and azotemia too was reversed.
It is *therefore* advisable that the patient continue bed rest.

Use a comma before and after Latin abbreviations (and their translations), such as *etc., i.e., e.g., et al., viz.,* when they are used as parenthetical expressions within a sentence.

See Latin abbreviations

participles
See
dangling modifiers
fused participles

particles in names
See personal names, nicknames, and initials

Patient "Bill of Rights"
A statement delineating certain rights of patients concerning their treatment, and in turn the behavior the patient is expected to exhibit related to therapy, followup, and conduct. Various such statements have been adopted by the American Hospital Association, professional groups, and individual institutions.

pc, p.c.
Abbreviation *pc* is for *photocopy* and *p.c.* is for *post cibum.*

See
copy designation
drug terminology

pct.
See percent

per
See virgule

percent (%)

Note that *percent* is a single word. Do not use the abbreviation *pct.* except in tables. Instead, use % or *percent*.

50% *or* fifty percent *not* 50 pct.

Use the symbol % after a numeral. Do not space between the numeral and the symbol.

13% monos, 1% bands
She has had a 10% increase in weight since her last visit.
MCHC 34%
10% solution

Use numerals for the number preceding % (except at beginning of sentence).

50% *not* fifty %

When the number is written out, write out *percent*.

Fifty percent of the patients were given a placebo.

When the amount is less than 1 percent, place a zero before the decimal.

0.5% *not* .5%

With whole numbers, avoid following the number by a decimal point and 0, since such forms are easily misread. The decimal point and 0 may be used if it is important to express exactness.

5% *not* 5.0%

Use decimals, not fractions, with percents.

0.5% *not* 1/2%

Repeat % (or *percent)* with each quantity.

Values ranged from 13% to 18%.
not Values ranged from 13 to 18%.

Fifty percent to eighty percent ...
not Fifty to eighty percent ...

Percent of takes a singular verb when the word following *of* is singular, a plural verb when it is plural.

Ninety percent of the body was burned.
Forty percent of the patients were in the control group.

Percent takes a singular verb when it stands alone (not followed by *of*).

Fifty percent is adequate.

According to the SI (International System of Measuring Units), it is common and acceptable for percents to be expressed as a fraction of one. MT experience would indicate that it is more common and acceptable for *percent* to be dropped in dictation (and thus in transcription). Use the expression dictated; do not convert.

polys 58% *or* polys 0.58 *or* polys 58
MCHC 34% *or* MCHC 0.34 *or* MCHC 34

percentage point
Percentage point is not the same as *percent*. Thus, a decrease from 10 percent to 5 percent is a decrease of 5 percentage points, or a decrease of 50 percent, not a decrease of 5 percent.

See
chemical nomenclature
International System of Measuring Units

periods
Periods are most commonly used to mark closure. They may also be used as a mark of separation.
Place a period at the end of a declarative sentence.

The patient's past medical history is unremarkable.

Place a period at the end of an imperative sentence that does not require emphasis. For emphasis, use an exclamation point.

*There's not much to be said about a period except
that most writers don't reach it soon enough.*
William Zinzer

Do not lift heavy objects.
Never lift heavy objects!

Do not use a period at the end of a parenthetical sentence within another sentence.

When I saw him on his return visit (Dr. Smith saw him on his initial visit), I was startled by the deterioration in his condition.

If a sentence terminates with an abbreviation (or other word) that ends with a period, do not add another period to end the sentence.

He takes Valium 5 mg q.a.m.
not He takes Valium 5 mg q.a.m..

Always place the period inside quotation marks.

The patient's response was emphatic: "I will never consent to the operation."

laboratory data
Separate values of unrelated tests by periods.

White count 5.9. Urine specific gravity 1.006.

decimal point
The period may serve as a decimal point.

1.34 g

See related topics, including
abbreviations
acronyms
brief forms
chemical nomenclature

credentials, professional
decimals, decimal units
degrees, academic
ellipsis points
formats
genus and species names
International System of Measuring Units
laboratory data and values
Latin abbreviations
lists
money
numbers
personal names, nicknames, and initials
pH
question marks
quotations, quotation marks
sentences
specific gravity
state, county, city, and town names and resident designations
units of measure

personal names, nicknames, and initials

Capitalize personal names.

Jocelyn Jenik

foreign names of persons

Follow the person's preference for spelling, capitalization, and spacing.

Capitalize or lowercase the foreign particles *de, du, di, d', le, la, l', van, von, ter,* etc., according to the person's preference. Check references for guidance. Use lowercase if unable to determine preference. When a lowercased particle begins a sentence, it must be capitalized.

We inserted a de Pezzer catheter,
but De Pezzer catheters were used.

a DeBakey procedure

initials

Use a period after each initial within a name, but do not use periods when initials replace a complete name.

Names are not always what they seem. The common Welsh name Bzxxllwcp is pronounced Jackson.
Mark Twain

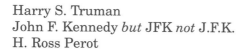

Harry S. Truman
John F. Kennedy *but* JFK *not* J.F.K.
H. Ross Perot

When an individual uses initials for first and middle names, do not space between them.

T.S. Eliot

Do not use a single initial with a last name unless it is the person's preference or you cannot determine the first name.

W. Madison

Jr, Jr.; Sr, Sr.
Abbreviations for *junior* and *senior* in names. Usage of a comma before and a period after is optional, but use both or neither. Do not use all capitals (JR, SR).

John F. Kennedy Jr
or John F. Kennedy, Jr.

name change
In the case of a name change, use both names until the new name is well known, then use only the new name.

Malcolm X
Mohammed Ali

nicknames
Do not use a nickname as the formal patient identifier unless the full name is not known. Otherwise, do not shorten a name or use a nickname unless that is the individual's clear preference. Do not enclose nicknames in quotation marks.

Patricia Forbis *as formal patient identifier, but otherwise* Pat Forbis

ordinals
Do not place a comma after a name and before an ordinal.

John D. Rockefeller III

personifications
Capitalize personifications, such as Mother Nature.

He kept saying, "You can't fool Mother Nature."

words derived from personal names
Do not capitalize words derived from personal names.

parkinsonism
cushingoid

See
eponyms
sex changes
titles

pII
Measure of acidity or alkalinity of a solution (e.g., urine or blood), ranging from 0 to 14, with 7 being neutral. Express by a whole number or a whole number followed by a decimal point and one or two digits. A whole number may be followed by a decimal point and 0 to demonstrate that the value following the decimal point has not been mistakenly deleted.
Do not express other than with a lowercased *p* and capital *H*. If the term begins a sentence, precede it by *The* or recast the sentence.

pH 7.55
pH 7.4
pH 7.0
The pH was 6.47.
not pH was 6.47.

pharmaceutical nomenclature
See drug terminology

phase

Lowercase *phase* and use arabic numerals.

phase 4

PhD

Abbreviation for *Doctor of Philosophy* degree. No periods, no spaces.

See degrees, academic

phrases

A phrase is a group of words without a subject and a verb. It usually begins with an adverb, preposition, or participle. Use a comma before and/or after a phrase when the sentence could be misread without it, but do not use such commas if they change the intended meaning. Follow the guidelines below.

The comma following a short opening adverbial phrase may be omitted. Use the comma for longer introductory phrases or when its absence might cause confusion.

Presently she is without pain.
During hospitalization, she will have a CAT scan.
Because of vomiting, an NG tube was put in place.

An introductory prepositional phrase is always correct with a following comma; it may be correct without one. Never omit the comma if it is needed for clarity. Introductory expressions in which the subject and verb are understood are clauses not phrases and should always be followed by a comma.

After surgery, he was taken to the recovery room.
If so, he will return sooner. (*If so* is understood to mean *if that is so.*)

Do not use a comma before or after other prepositional phrases unless it is needed for clarity.

The patient will return to my office *for continuing pain.*
The exam revealed a young white male *with multiple injuries.*

Do not use commas to set off essential participial phrases. Use commas to set off nonessential participial phrases.

Examination revealed two wounds *bleeding profusely* and several small bleeders.

The incision, *running from the umbilicus to the symphysis pubis,* was closed in layers.

The patient was admitted *screaming with pain.*

When a transitional phrase or independent comment occurs at the beginning of a second independent clause and it is preceded by a comma and *and, but, for, or, nor, yet,* or *so,* follow the transitional phrase with a comma.

He was improving, but in spite of physical therapy, he still had difficulty walking without assistance.

Phrases such as *in addition to, along with, as well as, together with,* and similar terms are not conjunctions, and they do not create a compound subject. So, they do not change a singular verb to a plural verb. Watch usage.

D: The patient, as well as his wife, were resistant to discussing alternative forms of treatment.

T: The patient, as well as his wife, was resistant to discussing alternative forms of treatment.

Note: If such terms are replaced by *and,* then they do create a compound subject and so there must be a plural verb. It is not appropriate, however, to make such a replacement.

The patient and his wife were resistant to discussing alternative forms of treatment.

See clauses

physical status classification
See classifications

physician
See doctor, physician

pico-
An inseparable prefix meaning one-trillionth of a unit. To convert to the basic unit, move the decimal point 12 places to the left.

5,678,123,456,891.4 picoseconds = 5.678123456891 seconds.

pint

dry pint
Equal to 33.6 cubic inches (one-half of a dry quart). Its metric equivalent is 0.55 liter. To convert to liters, multiply by 0.55.

liquid pint
Equal to 16 fluidounces or two cups. Its metric equivalent is 473 ml or 0.473 liter. To convert to liters, multiply by 0.473.

plain film x-rays
Not *plane* film.

Plain film of the abdomen was negative.

See plane

plane
An imaginary flat surface.
Planes of the body and its structures include the following. Check appropriate references for additional planes.

frontal	a vertical plane dividing the body or structure into anterior and posterior portions. Also known as coronal plane.
sagittal	lengthwise vertical plane dividing the body or structure into right and left portions; midsagittal plane divides the body into right and left halves. Also known as median plane.
transverse	plane running across the body parallel to the ground, dividing the body or structure into upper and lower portions. Also known as horizontal plane.

See plain film x-rays

planets
See heavenly bodies

plant names
Capitalize the first word in a botanical name. Lowercase other names of plants except the proper names or adjectives that are part of them.

Cannabis sativa
Her favorite flower is gardenia, but she is allergic to it.

plurals
Use the general rules to form plurals unless the dictionary provides the plural form. When the dictionary lists more than one plural form, the first is usually the preferred one. In general, do not use apostrophes to form plurals, but there are exceptions.

abbreviations
Add *s* (no apostrophe) following all-capital abbreviations.

WBCs *not* WBC's
EEGs *not* EEG's
PVCs *not* PVC's

Use *'s* to form the plural of lowercased abbreviations.

rbc's *not* rbcs

brief forms
Add *s* without an apostrophe.

exams
segs
polys

letters, symbols
Use *'s* to form the plural of single letters and symbols.

+'s
serial K's

medical terms derived from Latin or Greek
General rules follow. Consult appropriate medical dictionaries for additional guidance.

words ending in *en:* Change ending to *ina.*

foramen   foramina

words ending in *a:* Add *e.*

conjunctiva   conjunctivae

words ending in *us:* Change ending to *i.*

embolus   emboli

words ending in *on:* Change ending to *a.*

ganglion   ganglia

words ending in *is:* Change ending to *es.*

diagnosis   diagnoses

exceptions
arthritis   arthritides
epididymis   epididymides

words ending in *um:* Change ending to *a.*

diverticulum   diverticula

names (including eponyms)
Add *s* (or *es*) without an apostrophe to form the plural.

Babinskis were positive.
The Joneses were referred by ...

numbers, including years
Add *s* without an apostrophe. Exception: With single numerals, add *'s.*

500s
She is in her 20s.
6's and 7's.

units of measure, abbreviated
The singular and plural forms are the same. Do not add apostrophe or *s*.

5 mg
8 cc

special plural forms
Some words change form in the plural. Consult appropriate references for guidance.

singular	*plural*
child	children
woman	women

words that are always singular
Some words are always singular in usage.

ascites
herpes
lues

words that are always plural
Some words are always plural in usage.

adnexa
genitalia

words that may be singular or plural
Some words retain the same form, whether singular or plural.

biceps
facies
series

words that have alternative plural forms
Some words have more than one plural form. Use the preferred form. Consult appropriate references for guidance.

gases *preferred to* gasses

See specific entries, including the following:
abbreviations
acronyms
apostrophes
brief forms
compound words
eponyms
genus and species names
letters
numbers
symbols
units of measure

plus, plus sign (+)
Do not use the plus sign without a numeral.

+1, +2, +3, +4
or 1+, 2+, 3+, 4+
not +, ++, +++, ++++

in laboratory and technical readings
Use the symbol unless it will not be noticeable or clear.

3+ gram-positive cocci

meaning more than
Write out *plus* when it means more than.

At 40 plus, he considered himself old.

plus / minus
Express as *plus or minus* or *plus / minus,* not + / - except in tables.

See
positive sign
reflexes

p.m., PM
> *See*
> a.m., AM; p.m., PM
> time

p.o.
> *See* drug terminology

points of the compass
> *See* north, south, east, west

political divisions
> Include streets, cities, towns, counties, states, countries, etc.
>
> *See* geographic names

positional terms in anatomy
> *See* anatomic terms

positive findings
> Findings that are not normal. Opposite of negative or normal findings. Transcribe all findings, whether positive or negative.
>
> *See* negative findings

positive sign (+)
> Do not use except in special applications, e.g., blood nomenclature.
>
> blood type O+ *or* O positive
> Rh+ *or* Rh positive
>
> *See* plus, plus sign

possession

There are general and specialized rules for showing possession, as well as exceptions to these rules. Some of these rules and exceptions follow. Consult appropriate topics or references for specific applications.

nouns not ending with s
Show possession by adding *'s*.

patient's
children's
Jane's

nouns ending with s
For some, add *'s;* for others add an apostrophe only. Check references.

class's
physicians'

nouns as descriptive terms
Do not add an apostrophe to a noun ending in *s* when it is used as a descriptive term instead of a possessive. In proper names of this type, follow the user's practice.

educators conference
business leaders meeting
Veterans Administration
Doctors Hospital
Childrens Hospital (*entity does not use apostrophe in* Childrens)

eponyms
Do not use possessive form with eponymic terms.

Apgar score
Babinski sign
Down syndrome
Gram stain
Hodgkin disease

hyphenated compound terms
Use *'s* after the final word in hyphenated compound terms.

Her daughter-in-law's opinion was important to her.
Her sons-in-law's opinions did not interest her.

---

compound plurals containing a possessive
Keep the existing possessive term singular and make the second noun possessive, as well.

driver's licenses' renewal dates

individual possession, two or more individuals
Show possession after each name when possession is not joint.

Dr. Gray's and Dr. White's conclusions differed.

joint possession
Show possession only after the final name when possession is common to two or more individuals.

Drs. Smith and Brown's conclusion was ...

phrase or name combinations
Show possession only after the final word in phrase or name combinations.

Miller and Keane's reference
physician-in-chief's office

possessive pronouns
Do not use an apostrophe with possessive pronouns.

my conclusion
your referral
its course

units of time and money as possessive adjectives
Use *'s* or *s'*, whichever is appropriate. Do not confuse the possessive-adjective form with the compound-modifier form, which takes a hyphen.

one month's history *but* one-month history
three days' time *but* three-day time period
two cents' worth *but* two-cent piece

See
abbreviations
apostrophes
eponyms

money
pronouns
time

post meridiem
See a.m., AM; p.m., PM

Postal Service, postal service
Capitalize when referring to the US Postal Service. Lowercase generic uses.

See USPS guidelines

pound
Equal to 16 ounces (7000 grains). Equal to 454 grams (0.45 kilograms) in metric system. To convert to kilograms, multiply by 0.45. Abbreviation: lb. (with period).

Write out, do not use abbreviation (*lb.*) except in tables. Do not use a comma or other punctuation between units of the same dimension. Express with numerals.

12 pounds 13 ounces

prefixes
In most instances, do not use a hyphen to join most prefixes, including *ante-, anti-, bi-, co-, contra-, counter-, de-, extra-, infra-, inter-, intra-, micro-, mid-, non-, over-, pre-, post-, pro-, pseudo-, re-, semi-, sub-, super-, supra-, trans-, tri-, ultra-, un-, under-*. Common examples are noted below. Consult appropriate references for additional guidance.

antecubital
antithesis
bitemporal
cooperate
contraindication
counterproductive
defibrillate
extraterrestrial
infraumbilical

interpersonal
intracranial
microscope
midline
nontender
overenthusiastic
preoperative
posttraumatic
profile
pseudocele
reimburse
semicircular
sublingual
superficial
supramammary
transvaginal
trivalent
ultraviolet
unencumbered
underwear

for clarification
Use a hyphen after a prefix if it would have another meaning without the hyphen.

re-cover (*cover again*), recover (*regain*)
re-creation (*created again*), recreation (*playtime*)

Use a hyphen following a prefix to avoid an awkward combination of letters and when it will assist in reading and pronunciation.

re-x-rayed (but *x-rayed again* is preferred)
co-workers
re-emphasize

independent
Occasionally a prefix is used as an independent word.

Nodules were found in the left mid and lower lobes of the lung.
She is post L3 laminectomy.

self-
Use a hyphen with compounds with the prefix *self-*.

self-administered

with proper nouns, capitalized words, numbers, and abbreviations
Use a hyphen to join a prefix to a proper noun, capitalized word, number, or abbreviation.

pro-American
pre-1991 admission
non-Hodgkin-like lymphoma

with units of measurement
The metric system and SI units use prefixes to denote fractional or multiple units. These prefixes are joined without hyphens.

centimeter
milligram
kilogram

See
compound modifiers
compound words
hyphens
International System of Measuring Units
letters
numbers
suffixes
temperature, temperature scales
units of measure

preoperative and postoperative diagnoses
See diagnoses

prepositions
A preposition relates to its object, either a noun or a pronoun.

The patient was taken into the delivery room. (*Into* is the preposition; *the delivery room* is its object.)

common prepositions
about
across

after
against
along
among
around
at
before
below
beneath
beside
between
by
down
during
except
for
from
in
inside
into
like
near
of
off
on
outside
over
past
through
to
toward
under
underneath
until
up
with
within
without

Pronouns following prepositions must be in the objective case: *me, us, it, you, them.*

between you and me
not between you and I

I lately lost a preposition.
It hid, I thought, beneath my chair.
And angily I cried: 'Perdition!'
Up from out of in under there!
Marius Bishop

president-elect
Lowercase except when used as a formal title before a name (and even then, *elect* is lowercased). Hyphenate.

She is president-elect of AAMT.
They were introduced to President-elect Hurley.

prior to
See before, prior to

prioritize
A back-formation from *priority,* increasingly used and accepted. Transcribe if dictated.

We prioritized the events.

p.r.n.
See drug terminology

problem-oriented medical record
A system for patient care documentation that numbers a patient's problems (diagnoses, conditions) and describes and reports on them in an organized manner described as SOAP notes.

See
Appendix A, "Sample Reports"
SOAP notes

They didn't want it good, they wanted it Wednesday.
Robert Heinlein

productivity
The quantitative measure of work produced over a designated period of time. It is influenced by numerous factors, all of which must be taken into account and which vary from setting to setting.

While there is no such thing as a national productivity standard for medical transcription (nor can there be one), the productivity within an individual work setting can be measured.

Productivity standards, to be effective, must address quality as well as quantity.

Words should be weighed and not counted.
Yiddish proverb

For discussions on and guidelines for developing institutional standards on an individual basis, see the appendices noted below.

See
Appendix P, "Customizing Productivity Standards"
Appendix Q, "How Much Wood Should a Woodchuck (or a Medical
    Transcriptionist) Chuck?"
Appendix R, "The Q-P Zone"
Appendix S, "They're Asking the Wrong Questions"
Appendix T, "Transcription by the Pound"
quality of medical transcription
standard unit of measure for medical transcription

profanities
   See obscenities, profanities, vulgarities

professional credentials
   See credentials, professional

professional liability insurance
   Insurance covering most kinds of wrongful or negligent conduct an MT might conduct in his/her profession. It usually does not cover risks covered by property/casualty insurance and has other exclusions.
   There continues to be a diversity of views as to whether it is prudent for medical transcriptionists to carry professional liability insurance, a.k.a. errors and omissions insurance. Some states or employers require it for businesses providing medical transcription services, and some MT employees are seeking it because they are concerned about practices they are directed to perform that may subject them to liability risk, e.g., auto-authentication.
   AAMT anticipates offering a group plan that would be available both to individual medical transcriptionists and to services that employ MTs. For an update on its status, contact AAMT.

   See
   Appendix K, "Errors, Omissions, and the MT"
   Appendix B, "The Mark of Zorro"
   audit trails
   risk management

progress note
   An interim note in a patient's medical record, made by medical staff and other authorized personnel. Traditionally handwritten, more and more progress notes are dictated and transcribed.

   See Appendix A, "Sample Reports"

pronouns

personal
   Personal pronouns have person and number as well as subjective (S), possessive (P), and objective (O) forms.

	S	*P*	*O*
first person singular	I	mine	me
first person plural	we	ours	us
second person singular	you	yours	you
second person plural	you	yours	you
third person singular	he/she/it	his/hers/its	him/her/it
third person plural	they	theirs	them

The personal pronoun must agree in number and gender to the preceding noun or pronoun to which it refers.

The patient was sent to the postpartum floor. She improved steadily.

Do not use an apostrophe with possessive pronouns. In particular, be careful not to confuse *its* with *it's*. *Its* (no apostrophe) is the possessive form of *it*. *It's* is the contraction form of *it is*.

> my conclusion
> your referral
> his review of systems
> our plan
> its significance (*not* it's)
> ours *not* our's
> theirs *not* their's
> yours *not* your's

reflexive
Reflexive pronouns are pronouns combined with -*self* or -*selves*. They refer to and emphasize the subject of the verb.

She insisted on feeding herself.

relative
Relative pronouns (*that, who, whom, what, which,* and their variations *whoever, whomever, whosoever, whatever, whichever*) refer to previous nouns as they introduce subordinate clauses.
Use *who* or *whom* to introduce an essential clause referring to a human being or to an animal with a name. Use *that* or *which* to introduce an essential clause referring to an inanimate object or to an animal without a name. Exception: When *that* as a conjunction is used elsewhere in the same sentence, use *which*, not *that,* to introduce an essential clause. Do not use commas to set off essential subordinate clauses.

The patient came into the emergency room, and she was treated for
tachycardia that had resisted conversion in her physician's office.
He had two large wounds that were bleeding profusely and several
small bleeders.
She said that the dog which bit her was a miniature poodle.

Use *who* or *whom* to introduce a nonessential clause referring to a
human being or to an animal with a name. Use *which* to introduce a nonessential clause referring to an inanimate object or to an animal without
a name. Precede and follow the clause with a comma or closing punctuation.

The patient, who was referred by his family physician, came into the
emergency room.
The patient's parents, who had been summoned from Europe, were
consulted about her past history.

Take care of the sense, and the sounds will take care of themselves.
Lewis Carroll

without antecedents
Text with a pronoun that does not have a preceding noun or pronoun
should be edited to identify the pronoun's antecedent.

D *(first sentence of report):* She is a 40-year-old white female complaining of nausea and vomiting.
T: The patient is a 40-year-old white female complaining of nausea
and vomiting.

See clauses

pronunciation
It is not uncommon for medical transcriptionists to encounter mis-
pronunciations in dictation, in the classroom, and among themselves.
Of course, terms should be spelled correctly, not as they are pronounced.

D: perry ferry
T: periphery

D: diverticuli
T: diverticula

D: aeriation
T: aeration

See syllables

Proofread EVERYTHING, dummy!
Thomas "Wayne" Brazell

proofreading

Medical transcriptionists should proofread reports they transcribe. Proofreading should be done while transcribing, at the completion of transcription, and, when there is access to the printed copy, after printing the report.

For many MTs, there is no access to the printed report because it is printed remotely. In this circumstance, the MTs must perfect their on-screen proofreading skills both during and after completion of the transcript.

Spellcheckers and grammar checkers are supplements to, not replacements for, proofreading.

See
grammar
spellcheck, spellchecker

proper names, proper nouns
See
names
nouns

proportions
Always use numerals in expressions of proportions.

5 parts dextrose to 1 part water

proprietary name
See
drug terminology
names

providers' signatures
See
Appendix E, "AAMT Position Paper: Providers' Signatures"
authentication

provinces, Canadian
See Canada

publication titles
See titles

pulmonary and respiratory terms

breaths per minute, respirations per minute
Spell out. Do not abbreviate.

Respirations: 18 breaths per minute.
not Respirations: 18 bpm.

21 respirations per minute
not 21 rpm

Use virgules only in the following form. *See* virgule

Respirations: 21/min
but not
21 respirations/min

The following is abstracted from "Notes on Using this Word Book" in *Neonatology Word Book,* by Hazel Tank, CMT, and Catherine Gilliam, CMT (AAMT, 1991). For price information, contact AAMT.

primary symbols

Primary symbols used in pulmonary and respiratory terminology are the first terms of an expression and are expressed as follows:

C	blood gas concentration
P *or* p	pressure or partial pressure
Q	volume of blood
V	volume of gas
D	diffusing capacity
R	gas exchange ratio

secondary symbols for gas phase

Immediately follow the primary symbol. Express them as small capitals if possible; otherwise, use regular caps.

A *or* A	alveolar
B *or* B	barometric
E *or* E	expired
I *or* I	inspired
L *or* L	lung
T *or* T	tidal

secondary symbols for blood phase

Immediately follow the secondary symbol for gas phase. Express them as lowercased letters.

b	blood
a	arterial
c	capillary
v	venous

gas abbreviations

Usually the last element of the term. Express them as small capitals or regular capitals. Use subscripts for the numerals if available; otherwise, place them on-line.

CO_2 *or* CO_2 *or* CO2
O_2 *or* O_2 *or* O2
N_2 *or* N_2 *or* N2
CO *or* CO

physiology terms
Combine the above symbols for pulmonary and respiratory physiology terms.

PCO_2	partial pressure of carbon dioxide
$PaCO_2$	partial pressure of arterial carbon dioxide
PO_2	partial pressure of oxygen
PaO_2	partial pressure of arterial oxygen
V/Q	ventilation-perfusion ratio

punctuation
Follow punctuation rules and use punctuation to enhance the clarity and accuracy of the communication. Do not make exceptions without being able to justify doing so.

If not required by punctuation rules and not needed for clarity and/or accuracy, omit the punctuation. Consult specific entries and appropriate references for guidance.

See
apostrophes
colons
commas
dashes
ellipsis points
exclamation marks
hyphens
parentheses
periods
question marks
quotations, quotation marks
semicolons
sentences

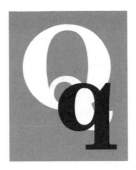

q., q.d., q.h., q.i.d., q.4h.
See drug terminology

quality assurance for medical transcription
Quality assurance for medical transcription contributes to risk management. AAMT's position paper on quality assurance in medical transcription outlines the appropriate expectations as well as the resources that are necessary to make those expectations appropriate and reasonable.

The tenets of total quality management are well suited to a quality assurance program for medical transcription.

See
Appendix U, "AAMT Position Paper: Quality Assurance Guidelines"
quality of medical transcription
risk management
total quality management

Quality is very simple. So simple, in fact,
that it is difficult for people to understand.
Roger Hale

quality of medical transcription
AAMT believes the quality of medical transcription is more important than its quantity. Without quality, the quantity matters little. High-quality medical transcription contributes to risk management.

See
Appendix F, "AAMT Explores Quality and Quantity Issues"
Appendix R, "The Q-P Zone"
Appendix U, "AAMT Position Paper: Quality Assurance Guidelines"
Appendix V, "Quality Assurance: Key to Cost Containment in Medical Transcription"
Appendix W, "The Quality of Patient Care Documentation"
productivity
quality assurance for medical transcription
risk management
total quality management

It is quality rather than quantity that matters.
Seneca

quantity
Use arabic numerals for quantities expressed with units of measure. Space between the quantity and the unit of measure.

4 mm

If a quantity begins a sentence, recast the sentence or write out both the quantity and the unit of measure.

See
numbers
units of measure

quantity of medical transcription
> *See*
> Appendix F, "AAMT Explores Quality and Quantity Issues"
> productivity
> quality of medical transcription
> standard unit of measure for medical transcription

quart
> Liquid measure equivalent to 2 pints or 32 fluidounces. Metric equivalent is approximately 950 milliliters or 0.95 liter. To convert to liters, multiply by 0.95.

question marks (?)

direct inquiry
> A question mark is used to indicate a direct inquiry. Thus, it is used at the end of an interrogative sentence (a direct question).

> Was the patient seen in the emergency room prior to admission?

indirect questions
> Use a period instead of a question mark at the end of indirect questions.

> The patient asked if he could be discharged by Saturday.

sentence including the word question
> Use a period instead of a question mark at the end of a declarative sentence that includes the word *question*.

> I question the consultant's conclusions.

polite requests in form of question
> Use a period instead of a question mark to end polite requests cast in the form of a question.

> Would you please change my appointment to Saturday.

> *Not knowing the question,*
> *It was easy for him*
> *To give the answer.*
> Dag Hammerskjold

question in form of declarative statement
Place a question mark at the end of a question in the form of a
declarative statement.

You mean you were serious when you said you smoke 50 cigarettes
a day?

question within a declarative sentence
Place a question mark at the end of a question that is part of a
declarative sentence.

How long will the operation take? I wondered.

series of incomplete questions
Place a question mark after each in a series of incomplete questions
that immediately follow and relate to a preceding complete question.

When was the patient last seen? Friday? Saturday? Sunday?

to express doubt or uncertainty
Use a question mark to indicate doubt or uncertainty. Sometimes,
particularly with diagnoses, a question mark is placed before a statement
in order to indicate uncertainty. Either placement is acceptable, but do
not place one both before and after.

His cholesterol levels were high normal (or minimally elevated?).

Diagnosis: Angina?
or Diagnosis: ?Angina
not Diagnosis: ?Angina?

with other punctuation
Place the question mark inside the ending quotation marks if the
material being quoted is in the form of a question. Follow "she said" or
similar attributions with a comma when they precede a quoted question.

The patient asked, "Must I return for followup that soon?"

Place the question mark outside the ending quotation mark if the quoted matter is not itself a question but is placed within an interrogative sentence.

Do you think he meant it when he said, "You'll be hearing from my attorney"?

Never combine a question mark with a comma, or with another ending punctuation mark, i.e., an exclamation mark, period, or other question mark. Thus, the question mark replaces the comma that normally precedes the ending quotation mark which is followed by "he said" or similar attributions.

"Are my symptoms serious?" she asked.

Place the question mark inside the closing parenthesis when the parenthetical matter is in the form of a question.

She said (did I hear correctly?) that she had five children, all delivered at home, and this is her first hospital admission.

Place the question mark outside the closing parenthesis when the parenthetical matter is not in the form of a question but is placed just prior to the end of an interrogative statement.

Did he return as scheduled for followup (the record is unclear)?

See quotations, quotation marks

quotations, quotation marks (" ")
Be sure to use quotation marks (" "), if available, instead of ditto marks (" "). Place quotation marks at the beginning and end of a quotation. If an uninterrupted quotation extends beyond one paragraph, place opening quotation marks at the beginning of each paragraph, but place an ending quotation mark only at the end of the final quoted paragraph.

capitalization
Begin a complete quotation with a capital letter if it is not grammatically joined to what precedes it.

Quoting: *The art of repeating erroneously the words of another.*
Ambrose Bierce

Path report reads, "Specimen is consistent with microadenoma."

Do not use a capital letter to begin incomplete quotations or those joined grammatically to what precedes them.

She says that she has "bad blood."

Capitalize the first word in a direct question even if the question is not placed within quotation marks.

She refused to answer the question, What is your name?

commas
Always place the comma following a quotation inside the closing quotation marks.

The patient stated that "the itching is driving me crazy," and she scratched her arms throughout our meeting.

periods
Always place periods inside quotation marks.

The consultant's report reads "The patient is a 21-year-old male referred to me by Dr. Wilson."

question marks
The placement of the question mark in relationship to ending quotation marks depends on the meaning. Place the question mark inside the ending quotation marks if the material being quoted is in the form of a question. Follow "she said" or similar attributions with a comma when they precede a quoted question. (Note that no period follows the quotation; never combine a question mark with a period.)

The patient asked, "Must I return for followup that soon?"

I hate quotations. Tell me what you know.
Ralph Waldo Emerson

Place the question mark outside the ending quotation mark if the quoted matter is not itself a question but is placed within an interrogative sentence.

Do you think he meant it when he said, "You'll be hearing from my attorney about this"?

semicolons
Place the semicolon outside the quotation marks.

The patient clearly stated "no allergies"; yet, his medical record states he is allergic to penicillin.

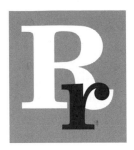

race
> *See* sociocultural designations

range
> Use numerals. It is acceptable to use a hyphen between the limits of a range if the following five conditions are met.

> 1. The phrases "from, to," "from, through," "between, and" are **not** used.
> 2. Decimals and/or commas do not appear in the numeric values.
> 3. Neither value contains four or more digits.
> 4. Neither value is a negative.
> 5. Neither value is accompanied by a symbol.

> When all five conditions are not met, use *to* in place of a hyphen. (*To* may be used, of course, even if the conditions are met.)

> 8-12 wbc *or* 8 to 12 wbc
> *but*
> $4 to $5 million dollars
> -25 to +48.
> Weight fluctuated between 120 and 130 pounds.
> Platelet counts: 120,000 to 160,000.

> Do not use a colon between the limits of a range. Colons are used to express ratios, not ranges.

> 80-125 *not* 80:125

ratio

The relationship of one quantity to another. The value is expressed with numerals separated by a colon. Do not replace the colon with a virgule, dash, hyphen, or other mark.

Mycoplasma 1:2
cold agglutinins 1:4
Zolyse 1:10,000
Xylocaine 1:200,000

Use *to* or a hyphen instead of a colon when the expression includes words or letters instead of values. Consult appropriate references for guidance.

I-to-E ratio
myeloid-erythroid ratio
FEV-FVC ratio

rbc, RBC

See blood counts

recur, recurrence, recurrent

Not *reoccur, reoccurrence, reoccurrent.*

The patient had recurring infections.
Diagnosis: Recurrent fever.

red blood cells, red blood count

See blood counts

redundancies

See expendable words

references

MTs need and use a variety of reference materials to assist them in preparing transcripts of medical dictation. At various points throughout this text, the reader is advised to consult appropriate references for guidance. It is impossible for us to identify which references are appropriate

Words fascinate me. They always have.
For me, browsing in a dictionary
is like being turned loose in a bank.
Eddie Cantor

for each topic, but we do advise that criteria for selecting appropriate references should include the qualifications of the author(s), and/or editor(s), and/or publisher. Publications by or promoted by medical associations related to a particular topic may be especially good resources.

Do not be surprised by inconsistencies within and among even the most appropriate and respected of publications. The medical and English languages, as well as the practice of medicine, are in constant development—and no author, editor, or publisher is perfect.

It is important for each medical transcription department or office to identify its preferred references in order to promote consistency among its MTs and within its reports. Of course, AAMT encourages that *The AAMT Book of Style for Medical Transcription* be among those preferred references. A department notebook citing preferred references and noting any departmental exceptions is recommended.

AAMT publishes the *MT Resource Library* annually in its journal (*JAAMT*) and provides a complimentary copy to each new AAMT member. This is a list of resources used by MTs; no recommendations or assessments are made. Contact the AAMT office (800-982-2182 or 209-551-0883; fax 209-551-9317) for price information for nonmembers and for multiple copies.

reflexes
Graded 0 to 4. Express as an arabic numeral followed (or preceded) by a plus sign (except 0 which stands alone).

grade	meaning
0	absent
+1 *or* 1+ *not* +	decreased
+2 *or* 2+ *not* ++	normal
+3 *or* 3+ *not* +++	hyperactive
4 *or* 4+ *not* ++++	clonus

Do not use plus signs without the numeral, i.e., do not use +, ++, +++, ++++.

See plus, plus sign

regular type

Also known as plain type, regular type is preferred throughout medical transcription, with just a few exceptions when italics or bold type may be preferred or required.

Use regular type for English and medical terms as well as for foreign words and phrases that are commonly used in the English language.

in toto
cul-de-sac
en masse
peau d'orange
bruit

Use regular type, as well, in the following instances even though italics may be called for in manuscript preparation.

names of foreign institutions and organizations
Latin names of genera and species
chemical elements
arbitrary designations: patient B
letters indicating shape: T-bar
abbreviations: AFB
musical notations: F minor

See
allergies
bold type
italics

release of information

Release of information from medical records involves both legal requirements and professional responsibility. MTs should not release information except as authorized by institutional policies and procedures, and consistent with the law. The patient's rights to personal and informational privacy and confidentiality must be respected. At the same time, courts and others may have legitimate rights to record information.

See
confidentiality
risk management

respiratory terms
See pulmonary and respiratory terms

respirations per minute
See pulmonary and respiratory terms

ribonucleic acid
See genetics terminology

ring accent mark (°)
See accent marks

All of life is management of risk,
not its elimination.
Walter Wriston

risk management
Healthcare institution activities that identify, evaluate, reduce, and prevent the risk of injury and loss to patients, visitors, staff, and the institution itself. Medical transcriptionists play an important role in risk management through their commitment to quality in medical transcription and through their alertness to dictated information that indicates potential risk to the patient or the institution, including its personnel. When identified, such information should be brought to the attention of the appropriate institutional personnel, identified in the institution's program policies.

Cross-references below address some of the topics that relate medical transcription to risk management.

> *See*
> audit trails
> authentication
> blank
> confidentiality
> date dictated, date transcribed
> derogatory and inflammatory remarks
> dictated but not read
> double entendres
> editing
> errors in dictation
> flag
> inconsistencies in dictation
> jargon
> obscenities, profanities, vulgarities
> professional liability insurance
> quality assurance for medical transcription
> quality of medical transcription
> release of information
> transcribed but not read
> verbatim transcription

RNA
See genetics terminology

roman numerals
See numbers

room names and numbers
See building, structure, and room names

root words
The main component of a term. Other parts include prefix, suffix, and combining vowel. The joining of a root word with its combining vowel creates the combining form.

gastrology =
gastr   root word
o   combining vowel
logy   suffix

endometritis =
endo   prefix
metr   root word
itis   suffix

rpm

Abbreviation meaning *revolutions per minute*. Do not use as abbreviation for *respirations per minute*.

30 respirations per minute, *not* 30 rpm

Rule of Nines

See classifications

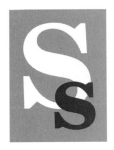

s̄
    Symbol for *without*. Frequently used in handwritten notes. Express in full in transcribed reports.

Saint, Sainte
    Abbreviation: *St.* (saint), *Ste.* (sainte). Use abbreviation in names of saints. Use full term or abbreviation in surnames and geographic names, according to preferred or common usage.

    Susan St. James
    St. Mary's Hospital
    St. Louis
    Sault Sainte Marie

salutation
    Greeting line in letters (Dear…). Use courtesy titles (Dr., Ms., etc.), followed by a colon or a comma, according to letter style and format you use.

    Note: While salutation lines continue to be the preferred and common practice, it is acceptable to drop them in form letters or in those instances when the appropriate courtesy title is not known, for example, when you cannot determine whether the person is male or female. *To Whom It May Concern* is another alternative in that instance, but it appears to be losing favor.

    See titles

"same"
See diagnoses

Saturday
See days of the week

scales
Use arabic numerals.

Ballard scale
A scoring system for assessing the gestational age of infants based on neuromuscular and physical maturity. Scores, expressed in arabic numerals, are converted to gestational age (in weeks).

score	age (weeks)
5	26
10	28
15	30
20	32
25	34
30	36
35	38
40	40
45	42
50	44

earthquake magnitude scale
A one-unit increase on the scale equals a tenfold increase in ground motion. Express with arabic numerals and decimal point.

She was injured in an earthquake measuring 6.6.

French scale
Sizing system for catheters, sounds, and other tubular instruments. Each unit is approximately 0.33 mm in diameter. Precede by # or *No.* if the word *number* is dictated.

5-French catheter
#5-French catheter
catheter, size 5 French

Keep in mind that *French* is linked to diameter size not to the instrument being measured. Thus, it is a 15-French catheter, not a French catheter, size 15.

Glasgow coma scale
Describes level of consciousness of patients with head injuries by testing the patient's ability to respond to verbal, motor, and sensory stimulation. Each parameter is scored on a scale of 1 through 5, then totals are added together to indicate level of consciousness. (Glasgow refers to Glasgow, Scotland.)

score	*level of consciousness*
14 or 15	normal
7 or less	coma
3 or less	brain death

Outerbridge scale
Assesses damage in chondromalacia patellae. Lowercase *grade,* and use arabic numerals 1 (minimal) through 4 (excessive).

Diagnosis: Chondromalacia patellae, grade 3.

See
cancer classifications
classifications
scores
temperature, temperature scales

scores
Most scoring systems use arabic numerals. Check appropriate references.

His IQ score is 118.

Apgar score
Assessment of newborn's condition in which pulse, breathing, color, tone, and reflex irritability are each rated 0, 1, or 2, at one minute and five minutes after birth. Each set of ratings is totaled, and both totals are reported. Named after Virginia Apgar, MD. Do not confuse with APGAR questionnaire.

Use initial capital only. Express ratings with arabic numerals. Write out the numbers related to minutes, so that attention is drawn to the scores.

Apgars 7 and 9 at one and five minutes.

Catterall hip score
Rating system for Legg-Perthes disease (pediatric avascular necrosis of the femoral head). Use roman numerals I (no findings) through IV (involvement of entire head).

Catterall hip score I *or* Catterall score I

Gleason score
Also known as Gleason tumor grade. *See* cancer classifications.

Kurtzke disability score
Two-part scoring system to evaluate patients with multiple sclerosis. Part one evaluates functional systems (pyramidal, cerebellar, brain stem, sensory, bowel and bladder, visual, mental, and other). Part two is a disability status scale from 0 to 10.

trauma score
Scoring system that measures systolic blood pressure, respiratory rate and expansion, capillary refill, eye opening, and verbal and motor responses on a scale of 2 through 16. Score predicts injury severity and probability of survival.

See
APGAR questionnaire
cancer classifications
classifications
scales

seasons
Do not capitalize the names of seasons unless they are part of a formal name.

spring
summer
autumn
fall

winter
Winter Olympics

self-
See prefixes

semiannual, semimonthly, semiweekly

semiannual
Occurring twice yearly; biannual. Do not confuse with *biennial* which means every other year.

semimonthly
Occurring twice monthly. Do not confuse with *bimonthly,* which means occurring every two months.

semiweekly
Occurring twice weekly. Do not confuse with *biweekly,* which means occurring every two weeks.

See biannual, biennial, bimonthly, biweekly

> ***Do not be afraid of the semicolon;***
> ***it can be most useful.***
> Ernest Graves

semicolons
In general, use a semicolon to mark a separation when a comma is inadequate and a period is too final.

independent clauses
Use a semicolon to separate closely related independent clauses when they are not connected by a conjunction (*and, but, for, nor, yet, so*). Alternatively, the independent clauses may be written as separate sentences,

but keep in mind that the semicolon demonstrates a relationship or link between the independent clauses that the period does not.

> The patient had a radical mastectomy for a malignancy of the breast; the nodes were negative. *(preferred)*
> *or* The patient had a radical mastectomy for a malignancy of the breast. The nodes were negative. *(acceptable)*

Use a semicolon before a conjunction connecting independent clauses if one or more of the clauses contain complicating internal punctuation.

> The left inguinal region was prepped and draped in the usual fashion; and with 2% lidocaine for local anesthesia, a radiopaque #4 French catheter was introduced into the left common femoral artery, employing the Seldinger technique.

Use a semicolon to separate closely related independent clauses when the second begins with a transitional word or phrase such as *also, besides, however, in fact, instead, moreover, namely, nevertheless, rather, similarly, therefore, then,* or *thus.* Alternatively, the independent clauses may be written as separate sentences, but again, keep in mind that the semicolon shows a link or relationship between the clauses that the period does not.

> The patient had a radical mastectomy for a malignancy of the breast; however, the nodes were negative. *(preferred)*
> *or* The patient had a radical mastectomy for a malignancy of the breast. However, the nodes were negative. *(acceptable)*

items in a series

Use a semicolon to separate items in a series if one or more items in the series include other internal punctuation. This usage is frequently seen in lists of medications and dosages, as well as in lists of lab results.

> The patient received Cerubidine 120 mg daily x 3 on February 26, 27, and 28; he received Cytosar 200 mg IV over 12 hours x 14 doses beginning February 26; and thioguanine 80 mg in the morning and 120 mg in the evening x 14 doses, for a total dose of 200 mg a day, starting February 26.

> His lab results showed white count 5.9, hemoglobin 14.6, hematocrit 43.1; PT 11.2, PTT 31.4; and urine specific gravity 1.006, pH 6, with negative dipstick and negative microscopic exam.

quotations

In quotations, place the semicolon outside the quotation marks.

The patient clearly stated "no allergies"; yet, his medical record states he is allergic to penicillin.

See
clauses
elliptical constructions
quotations, quotation marks
sentences

senior

Lowercase in references to academic class and member of class.

She is a senior at Memorial High.
The senior class graduates Saturday.

Sr., Sr
See personal names, nicknames, and initials

senior citizen

While a patient's age may be relevant, ageist labels such as this should be avoided.

To me, old age is fifteen years older than I am.
Bernard M. Baruch

sentences

Use sentences to separate complete thoughts. Occasionally, a dictator will dictate a report as a single sentence or just a few sentences. Break the report up into appropriate sentences, paragraphs, and sections.

Capitalize the first letter of each sentence (including clipped sentences or sentence fragments). Do not begin a sentence with a word that must never be capitalized; instead, edit lightly or recast the sentence.

A perfectly healthy sentence is extremely rare.
Henry David Thoreau

The patient was referred by Dr. Watson.
Abdomen soft, nontender. Bowel sounds active.
Leads aVL and aVR were …

D: pH was 7.18.
T: The pH was 7.18.

clipped
    Complete sentences are the grammatically correct form, but physicians often dictate clipped sentences, omitting subjects, verbs, articles, as the case may be. The dictator may prefer that these clipped sentences be transcribed as dictated rather than edited to complete sentences. Dictated clipped sentences are acceptable when they achieve directness and succinctness without loss of clarity.

    Abdomen benign. Pelvic not done. Rectal negative.

    Clipped sentences are particularly prevalent and acceptable in surgical reports, laboratory data, review of systems, and the physical examination, even when complete sentences are used in the remaining sections of the report. Such a mix is acceptable.
    When the dictator's style is to dictate in clipped sentences (throughout the report or in certain sections), it is not necessary to expand dictated clipped sentences into complete sentences unless that is the dictator's preference.
    When an occasional clipped sentence appears within a report (or within a section of a report), it may be expanded into a complete sentence in order to make the report (or section) consistent, provided the change is not too extensive. Likewise, when an occasional complete sentence appears amidst clipped sentences, it may be clipped for consistency.

simple
    A simple sentence has a subject and a predicate (each can be singular or plural) expressing a single complete thought. It may also include multiple adjectives, adverbs, phrases, and appositives.

End each sentence with the appropriate ending punctuation (period, question mark, exclamation point).

The patient was placed on the operating table.

When there are only two subjects, do not separate them by punctuation. When there are more than two subjects, use series punctuation.

Pacemaker wires and mediastinal drainage tubes were inserted.

The aryepiglottic folds, arytenoids, and postcricoid space were normal.

When there are only two predicates, do not separate them by punctuation. When there are more than two predicates, use series punctuation.

He continued to improve and was discharged home on the second postoperative day.

He uses a lot of big words, and his sentences run from here back to the airport.
Carolyn Chute

compound
A compound sentence has two or more independent (but closely related) clauses, each of which could stand alone as a simple sentence; it may be joined by a comma and a conjunction (e.g., *and, but*) or by a semicolon.

Separate coordinate independent clauses joined by a coordinating conjunction (*and, but, or, nor*), by a comma, or by a semicolon if one of the clauses already contains punctuation and the semicolon will enhance clarity.

A sector iridotomy was done, and Zolyse was instilled.

When coordinate independent clauses are very short and closely related, they may be joined without a comma or semicolon.

The x-rays were normal and the gallbladder was well visualized.

Use semicolons to separate coordinate independent clauses that are not joined by a coordinating conjunction.

The specimen was sent to the pathologist for examination; he found nothing suspicious for carcinoma.

Conjunctive adverbs (*consequently, however, moreover, nevertheless, otherwise, therefore, thus*) are used between independent clauses. Precede them by a semicolon (sometimes a period), and follow them by a comma.

The patient remained febrile; nevertheless, he left the hospital against medical advice.
The pathologist found nothing suspicious for carcinoma on gross examination; however, frozen section demonstrated fibrocystic disease.

You can be a little bit ungrammatical if you come from the right part of the country.
Robert Frost

complex
A complex sentence has one independent (main) clause and one or more dependent (subordinate) clauses, which together express one complete thought.
Use a comma after a subordinate clause that precedes the main clause.

Although it was inflamed, the gallbladder was without stones.

compound-complex
A compound-complex sentence has two or more independent clauses and one or more dependent clauses.

The posterior pack was removed, and after the wound was copiously irrigated, the procedure was terminated.

See
clauses
conjunctions
editing
phrases
punctuation

September
See months

serial numbers
See equipment terms

series
Use a comma to separate a series of three or more items. Using a final comma before the conjunction preceding the last term is optional unless its presence or absence changes the meaning. (AAMT's practice is to use the final comma.)

Ears, nose, and throat are normal. *(final comma optional)*
No dysphagia, hoarseness, or enlargement of the thyroid gland. *(final comma required)*
The results showed blood sugar 46%, creatinine and BUN normal. *(no comma after* creatinine*)*

units of measure
Do not repeat units of measure in a related series.

140, 135, and 58 cc

colon
Sometimes, a colon (:) is used to introduce a series. *See* horizontal series *below.*

semicolon
Use semicolons, not commas, to separate items in a complex series or in a series in which one or more entries contain commas.

The patient was discharged on the following regimen: Carafate 1 mg four times a day, 30 minutes after meals and one at bedtime; bethanechol 25 mg p.o. q.i.d.; and Reglan 5 mg at bedtime on a trial basis.

horizontal series
Capitalize the first letter of each item in a horizontal series following a colon when the items are separated by periods. Lowercase the first letter of each item in a horizontal series following a colon when the items are separated by commas.

The patient's past medical history includes the following: Chronic silicosis. Status post left thoracotomy. Arteriosclerotic cardiovascular disease. Mild chronic seizure disorder.
but The patient's past medical history includes the following: chronic silicosis, status post left thoracotomy, arteriosclerotic cardiovascular disease, mild chronic seizure disorder.

parentheses
To avoid clutter and confusion, use parentheses instead of commas or em dashes to set off a series that describes what precedes it and that has internal commas. A colon is another alternative to the em dash when this type of series ends the sentence.

The patient had multiple complaints (headache, nausea, vomiting, and fever) and demanded to be seen immediately.
preferred to The patient had multiple complaints—headache, nausea, vomiting, and fever—and demanded to be seen immediately.

The patient had multiple complaints: headache, nausea, vomiting, and fever.
or The patient had multiple complaints (headache, nausea, vomiting, and fever).
preferred to The patient had multiple complaints—headache, nausea, vomiting, and fever.

unparallel series
Also known as *bastard enumeration* or *A, B, 3.* Correct an unparallel series by eliminating the serial-comma construction or editing the faulty portion to allow for serial-comma construction.

D: She had fever, chills, and was dyspneic.
T: She had fever and chills and was dyspneic.
or She had fever, chills, and dyspnea.

vertical series
    In a vertical series, capitalize the first letter of each entry, whether or not numbered; lowercase other words (except those that are always capitalized). End each entry with a period.

FINAL DIAGNOSES
1. Adult-onset diabetes mellitus.
2. Gastroenteritis.

See
colons
formats
lists
outlines
parellel construction

sex change

    Use the name and gender existing at the time referenced. Thus, if referring to the person before the operation, use the individual's name and gender at that time. If referring to the person after the operation, use the new name and gender.

sexist language

    Use sex-neutral terms unless a particular person is being referenced.
    Avoid creating new terms, e.g., *shem, shim.* Instead, use *he or she, him or her, his or her(s). S/he, he/she, him/her, his/her, his/hers* are increasingly used and acceptable, but their overuse leads to clutter, so wherever possible, edit to a plural pronoun or a sex-neutral noun.
    Use of plural pronouns with singular indefinite antecedents is increasingly used and is becoming more widely accepted, but purists continue to avoid it.

Everyone reported their findings.
or Everyone reported his or her findings.

    Where easily done, convert sexist nouns and adjectives to sex-neutral terms.

chairman *becomes* chair *or* chairperson
policeman *or* policewoman *becomes* police officer
businessmen *becomes* businesspersons

See age referents

shall, will

The usage distinctions between *shall* and *will* are lessening except in legal documents. Transcribe as dictated.

shorthand

A means of entering a term, phrase, or clause (or multiples thereof) with fewer keystrokes than character-by-character entry. Beware of shorthand entries that are words in their own right, or you may make mistakes similar to the following.

Dear Paroxysmal Atrial Tachycardia *when* Dear Pat *was intended.*

Modesto, Carcinoma *when* Modesto, CA *was intended.*

should, would

Should expresses obligation; *would* expresses usual action.
Use *would* in conditional past tense.

He should not continue smoking.
He would light up a cigarette automatically after meals.
If he had not smoked for so many years, it would not be so difficult
    for him to quit.

SI

Abbreviation for International System of Measuring Units (Système International d'Unités).

SI units

Units of measure associated with International System of Measuring Units.

See International System of Measuring Units

sic

Latin term meaning *so, thus, in this manner.* Use to show that you are repeating an error from the original, that you recognize it is an error, and that you did not make the error yourself.

Use lowercased letters without periods, and place term in brackets immediately following the error.

She said that voice recognition will eliminate third parties "like transcribers" [sic].

signature block

See
formats
titles

since

See because, due to, since

size

Lowercase *size.* Use arabic numerals.

size 8 shoes

*Slang is a language that rolls up its sleeves,
spits on its hands, and goes to work.*
Carl Sandburg

slang

In general, avoid slang terms and phrases except when they are essential to the report, when they more accurately communicate the meaning than their translation would, or when their meaning cannot be determined.

H. influenzae *not* H. flu
dexamethasone *not* dex
appendectomy *not* appy
tracheal, tracheostomy, *or* tracheotomy *not* trach

See
editing
jargon

slash (/)
Also known as *diagonal, solidus, or virgule.*

See virgule

smoking history
See pack-year history of smoking

so

When *so* means *so that,* introducing a clause describing purpose or outcome, it should not be preceded by a comma. It is acceptable, indeed preferred, in such instances to change *so* to *so that.*

D: He wanted to improve so he could attend his daughter's wedding.
T: He wanted to improve so that he could attend his daughter's wedding.
preferred to He wanted to improve so he could attend his daughter's wedding.

When *so* indicates *therefore,* precede *so* by a comma if it introduces a new independent clause. It is acceptable in such instances to change *so* to *and so.*

D: His condition was improved so he could attend his daughter's wedding.
T: His condition was improved, and so he could attend his daughter's wedding.
or His condition was improved, so he could attend his daughter's wedding.

SOAP notes

A prescribed format for patient care documentation. Acronym stands for:

S   subjective (patient's descriptions)
O   objective (clinician's observations)
A   assessment (clinician's interpretations)
P   plan (clinician's treatment plan)

See
Appendix A, "Sample Reports"
problem-oriented medical record

Social Security number

Nine-digit number assigned by Social Security Administration. It is grouped and hyphenated as follows:

030-34-5665

I've made it a point never to learn my Social Security number because I'm a person, not a number.
H. Ross Perot

sociocultural designations

Capitalize the names of languages, peoples, races, religions, political parties, but specify them only if pertinent, as in descriptive remarks to assure patient identification.

Hispanic
Filipino
Methodist
Caucasian

Color designations of race are usually not capitalized. However, *Black* is an acceptable sociocultural designation (*black* is also acceptable). Never capitalize *white*.

African American or *African-American* is an increasingly common sociocultural designation, preferred by many to *Black.* The noun form of *African American* may be hyphenated or not, but be consistent.

Do not substitute one race designation for a dictated (and acceptable) designation.

D: black *(without indication whether to capitalize or not)*
T: Black *or* black *not* African-American

D: white
T: white *not* White *not* Caucasian

Do not use derogatory or inflammatory terms except in direct quotations that are essential to the report. Bring inappropriate usage to the attention of those responsible for risk management.

See
derogatory and inflammatory remarks
nationalities

solidus (/)
Also known as *diagonal, slash,* or *virgule.*

See virgule

solutions
A normal solution, or molar solution, has a concentration equivalent to a gram-equivalent weight (mole) of solute per liter.

Express solution concentrations in relation to normality as follows:

normal	N
half normal	0.5N or N/2
twice normal	2N

D: half-normal saline
T: 0.5N saline
or N/2 saline
or half-normal saline

Express molarity as follows:

molar	mol/L
millimolar	mmol/L
micromolar	µmol/L

soundalikes
Terms that sound like other terms. Be alert so that you don't confuse such terms.

The patient was seen one day ago.
not The patient was seeing Juan Diego.

A re-injury was suffered when …
not Every injury was suffered when …

There are similar problems with interpreting look-alike terms.
Read "Look-alikes and Soundalikes" column in *Journal of AAMT* for both an educational and humorous look at these phenomena.

See look-alikes

How forcible are right words.
Job 6:25

south, southern, South, Southern
See north, south, east, west

spacing
See character spacing

Spanish names
Usual sequence is given name, father's family name, mother's family name, in that order. On second reference, drop the mother's family name

or use both, depending on individual's preference. If preference is not known, use both.

first reference: Juan Lopez Martinez
second reference: Juan Lopez *or* Juan Lopez Martinez

Some individuals use a *y* (meaning *and*) between the two family names. Use the *y* on second reference only if both names are used; otherwise, drop it.

first reference: Juan Lopez y Martinez
second reference: Juan Lopez *or* Juan Lopez y Martinez

A married woman may use her father's family name followed by *de* and her husband's name. Use just the husband's name on second reference.

first reference: Maria Perez de Martinez
second reference: Maria Martinez

species
    See genus and species names

specific gravity
    Express with four digits and a decimal point placed between the first and second digits.

specific gravity 1.020

speed
    Use numerals followed by appropriate abbreviation (or extended form if abbreviated form is not known or not commonly used).

80 rpm
65 mph

Machines should work. People should think.
John Peers

spellcheck, spellchecker
    Electronic spellcheckers are supplements, not replacements, for the medical transcriptionist's responsibility to proofread documents and assure that terms within them are spelled correctly. Look-alike terms will pass the scrutiny of spellcheckers as will other wrong words that are spelled accurately. Typographical errors that create real words will also be missed by the spellchecker.

    See
    proofreading
    spelling

spelling
    The cardinal rule of spelling in medical transcription is to use appropriate dictionaries and other references to determine the correct spelling of both medical and English terms. Do not accept the spelling offered by the dictator (or anyone else) unless you already know it is correct.
    Some words, English and medical, have more than one acceptable spelling. Use the preferred spelling, i.e., the spelling that accompanies the meaning in the dictionary, or if both accompany the meaning, the one listed first. Secondary spellings direct the reader to the preferred spelling for the meaning.
    When there is a discrepancy between the spelling in the medical dictionary and that in the English dictionary, use the medical spelling. For example, *Dorland's* gives no alternate spelling for *distention,* but *Webster's* gives *distension* or *distention.* In medical reports, then, use *distention.*
    Some idiosyncrasies will be encountered. For example, while *Dorland's* prefers *disk* to *disc,* when the root word is connected to a suffix, it is sometimes *disk-,* sometimes *disc-.* And, although *curet* is preferred to *curette,* the double-t form must be used in word forms derived from the root term.

    diskectomy *not* discectomy
    discogenic *not* diskogenic
    curet *but* curetting, curetted, curettage

> *My spelling is Wobbly. It's good spelling but it Wobbles, and letters get in the wrong place.*
> A.A. Milne

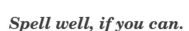

> *Spell well, if you can.*
> Lucy Hay

See
alternative acceptable forms
Appendix Y, "Medical Language"
editing
references

split verbs, split infinitives
    See verbs

spring
    See seasons

squinting modifiers
    See adverbs

Sr., Sr
    See personal names, nicknames, and initials

St., Ste.
    See Saint, Sainte

stage
Do not capitalize.

See cancer classifications

standard time
See time zones

standard unit of measure for transcription
There is no standard unit of measure for medical transcription. Units used include bits, bytes, characters, words, lines, pages, reports, minutes of dictation. AAMT encourages the use of clear, consistent definitions, where possible, and prefers the character as the basic unit of measure, where such measures are appropriate. However, AAMT recognizes that quality counts more in medical transcription than does quantity.

See
Appendix F, "AAMT Explores Quality and Quantity Issues"
productivity
quality of medical transcription

*It is not the quantity, but the pertinence
[of your words] that does the business.*
Seneca

state, county, city, and town names and resident designations

abbreviations
Do not abbreviate state names in text when they stand alone. State names may be abbreviated in text when they are accompanied by a city or town name; traditional state abbreviations continue to be used, but two-letter US Postal Service abbreviations are increasingly acceptable. Use US Postal Service state abbreviations in addresses.

Do not use a period after the two-letter state abbreviations approved by the US Postal Service. Use a period after traditional state abbreviations.

She flew here from Oregon yesterday.
not She flew here from Ore. yesterday.

He was admitted to Cook County Hospital in Chicago, IL.

MA
Mass.

Do not abbreviate county, city, or town names in text or in addresses.

New York City *not* NYC

capitalization
Always capitalize the initial letter of a state, county, city, or town name or a resident designation.

Boston, Massachusetts
Bostonian

Lowercase the phrase *county of* unless referring to a county's government. Lowercase generic uses, including use as an adjective to refer to a level of government.

The county of Stanislaus includes Modesto, California.
The County of Stanislaus held a budget hearing.
Assessment of county highways …

Lowercase the phrase *state of* unless referring to a state's government. Lowercase generic uses, including use as an adjective to refer to a level of government.

The state of California has many geographies.
The State of California challenged the federal mandate.
state coffers
state highways

Lowercase the phrase *city of* unless referring to a city's government. Lowercase generic uses, including use as an adjective to refer to a level of government. The same guidelines apply to *town, village,* etc.

The city of Modesto is growing.
The City of Modesto challenged the state mandate.
The city budget ...
The town of Ceres is contiguous to Modesto, California.
The Town of Ceres challenged the county mandate.

Capitalize *city* or similar term only if an integral part of an official name, commonly used name or nickname, or in official references. Otherwise, lowercase. The same guidelines apply to *town, village,* etc.

New York City
City of Commerce (official name of city)
the Windy City
The town budget was reviewed.

In titles, capitalize *city* or similar term only if part of a formal title placed before a name; lowercase when not part of a formal title or when the title follows the name. The same guidelines apply to *town, village,* etc.

City Manager Dixon
William Howard, city supervisor
Alfreda Noel, town councilperson

commas
Follow city or town name by a comma, then state or country name unless the city or town name can stand alone.

Modesto, California
Venice, Italy
San Francisco
Boston

Place a comma before and after the state name preceded by a city or county name, or a country name preceded by a state or city name.

The patient moved to Dallas, Texas, 15 years ago.
The patient returned from a business trip to Paris, France, the week
    prior to admission.

In addresses, place a comma after the city name but not after the state name.

Modesto, CA 95357

Place a comma between the county name and the state name.

Worcester County, Massachusetts

resident designations
    See spelling *below.*

spelling
    Follow the spelling in the US Postal Service Directory of Post Offices.
Use Appendix CC as a reference for state names, abbreviations (standard
and USPS), major cities by state, and state/city resident designations.

ZIP codes and state abbreviations
    In a mailing address, capitalize both letters of the two-letter state
abbreviation, and place a single space (no comma) between the state
abbreviation and the ZIP code. Use a hyphen or en dash between the
first five and last four digits of a ZIP-plus-four code.

Modesto, CA 95357
Modesto, CA 95357-6187

See
Appendix CC, "State Names and Abbreviations, Major Cities, and
    State/City Resident Designations"
geographic names
USPS guidelines

station
    See obstetrics terminology

status post
    Latin phrase meaning state or condition after or following. Do not
italicize. Do not hyphenate. Do not join *post* to the word or phrase following it.

status post hysterectomy
status post TIA

sterilely
    This is the only correct spelling.

street names and numbers

When part of a formal street name, spell out such terms as *street, avenue, boulevard, road, drive* within the narrative portions of reports and letters. Abbreviate and capitalize such terms in the address portion of a letter or on an envelope (St., Ave., Blvd., Rd., Dr.), using all capitals and no periods on envelope addresses (ST, AVE, BLVD, RD, DR). Do not abbreviate similar but less commonly used terms, e.g., *alley, lane,* in any instance, including the address portion of a letter or envelope.

> JOHNSON STROTHERS
> 1408 SUTTER ST
> MODESTO CA 95353
> *but*
> Johnson Strothers lives at 1408 Sutter Street, Modesto, California.
> He lives on Sutter Street.

When used alone (without a name) or following more than one name, spell out and lowercase all such terms.

> She lives down the street from the hospital.
> He lives at Hyde and Sutter streets.

numbered streets

Spell out and capitalize *First* through *Ninth;* use numeric ordinals for 10th and higher.

> He lives on Third Street.
> She lives on 23rd Avenue.

Abbreviate compass points to indicate directional ends of a street or city quadrants in a numbered address. Do not use periods. Do not precede by a comma.

> 1500 Pennsylvania NW

For decades of numbered streets, use figures and add *s,* no apostrophe.

> the 40s, the 1400s, etc.

See
addresses
geographic names
USPS guidelines

structures, monuments, etc.
　　See building, structure, and room names

style
　　See "Introduction"

> ***Proper words in proper places,***
> ***make the true definition of a style.***
> Jonathan Swift

subheadings
　　See formats

subject-verb agreement
　　See verb-subject agreement

subordinate conjunctions
　　See conjunctions

subscripts
　　Use subscripts only if your equipment places them appropriately and in reduced size; otherwise, place the character(s) on-line or use an alternative form.

　　CO_2 *or* CO2 *or* carbon dioxide

suffixes
　　Some suffixes are joined directly to the root word they refer to, others are joined by a hyphen, and still others remain separated by a character space. General guidelines follow. Consult appropriate medical and English dictionaries for additional guidance.

Join most suffixes directly to the root word (without a hyphen), including *-fold, -hood, -less, -wise.* Consult an appropriate dictionary for guidance.

likelihood
likewise
nevertheless
threefold

Sometimes, use a hyphen to avoid triple consonants or vowels.

shell-like
ileo-ascending colostomy

numbers and letters
Use a hyphen to join most compound nouns with a number or single letter as a suffix; in other instances, separate them by a space. Check appropriate references for specific terms.

vitamin D
factor V
Billroth II anastomosis

independent usage
Occasionally, a suffix is used as an independent word.

The abdomen exhibits no megaly.
Lysis of adhesions was done.

See
hyphens
prefixes

summer
See seasons

Sunday
See days of the week

super-, supra-

Super- means more than, above, superior, or in the upper part of the term to which it is joined. *Supra-* means in a position above the part of the term to which it is joined (in this sense, then, the same as *super-*).

Although *super-* may mean the same as *supra-,* the two are not generally interchangeable. Check appropriate references for guidance as to correct prefix. Both prefixes are generally joined directly to the following term, but the usual exceptions apply.

superego
supernatant
supraglottic
supraorbital
Super Tuesday
Superman

See prefixes

superscripts

Use superscripts only if your equipment places them appropriately and in reduced size; otherwise, place the character(s) on-line or use an alternative form.

33 m^2 *or* 33 sq m

surgical procedure report

See operative report

surnames

See
personal names, nicknames, and initials
Spanish names

suspensive hyphenation

See hyphens

suture sizes

Brown and Sharp gauge (B&S gauge)
System for sizing stainless steel sutures. Use whole numbers ranging from 40 (smallest) to 20 (largest). Thus, a size 30 suture is smaller than a size 25.

USP system
Sizes steel sutures and sutures of other materials. Sizes range from 11-0 (smallest) to 7 (largest). Thus, a size 7 suture is different from and larger than a size 7-0 suture.

Use 0 or 1-0 for single-aught suture; use the "digit hyphen zero" style to express sizes 2-0 through 11-0. Express sizes 1 through 7 with whole numbers. Place the symbol # before the size if "number" is dictated.

1-0 nylon *or* 0 nylon
2-0 nylon *not* 00 nylon
4-0 Vicryl *not* 0000 Vicryl
#7 cotton *not* 0000000 cotton

> ### A great many people think that polysyllables are a sign of intelligence.
> Barbara Walters

syllables
Division of words based on and guiding accurate pronunciation. Beware of extra syllables that slip into dictation. Transcribe words as they should be spelled, not as they are pronounced.

D: aeriation
T: aeration

See
pronunciation
word division

symbols

Use 's to form the plural of most symbols.

+'s
serial K's

See specific entries, including
ampersand
c̄
chemical nomenclature
degrees
division symbol
equal, equal to
greater than
Greek letters
International System of Measuring Units
less than
minus, minus sign
negative sign
No., #
numbers
percent
plus, plus sign
positive sign
s̄
virgule
x

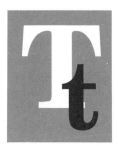

T

transcribed
    T as abbreviation for *transcribed* is used throughout this text to indicate the transcribed text in contrast to that dictated (*D*).

electroencephalographic electrodes
    T refers to temporal electrodes. Use subscripted numerals if available. Otherwise, place them on-line.

    T_3, T_4 midtemporal electrodes
    T_5, T_6 posterior temporal electrodes

heart sounds
    T refers to tricuspid valve. Use subscripted numerals if available. Otherwise, place them on-line.

    T_1 tricuspid valve component

lymphocytes
    Do not hyphenate noun forms, but do hyphenate adjective forms.

    T lymphocytes *but* T-lymphocyte count
    T cells *but* T-cell count

thyroid hormones
    Use subscripted numerals if available. Otherwise, place them on-line.

    triiodothyronine T_3 *or* T3
    thyroxine T_4 *or* T4

TNM tumor staging system
T refers to tumor size or involvement. Place the numerals on-line.

T2, N1, M1

vertebra
T refers to a thoracic vertebra. Place the numerals on-line.

T1 through T12

See
cancer classifications
cardiology terminology
electroencephalographic terms
hormones
lymphocyte and monoclonal antibody nomenclature
vertebra

tables, tabular matter

Tables are formatted presentations of tabular matter, separate from the narrative presentation in a report. Abbreviations not generally acceptable elsewhere may be used in such tabular matter provided they are readily recognizable.

tablespoon

Equal to three teaspoons or one-half of a fluidounce. Metric equivalent is approximately 15 milliliters. To convert to millilters, multiply by 15. Abbreviations: T, tbs., tbs, tbsp., tbsp

tablespoonful
Plural: *tablespoonfuls*

take

See bring, take

teaspoon

Equal to one-third of a tablespoon, one and one-third fluidram, or one-sixth of a fluidounce. Metric equivalent is approximately 5 milliliters. To convert to milliliters, multiply by 5. Abbreviations: t, tsp., tsp

teaspoonful
Plural: *teaspoonfuls*

telephone numbers

In the local 7-digit number, place a hyphen between the 3rd and 4th digits. Place the 3-digit area code and a hyphen before the 7-digit telephone number instead of in parentheses. Note: En dashes may be used instead of hyphens.

800-982-2182 or 800–982–2182
preferred to (800) 982-2182

temperature, temperature scales

It is meaningless to say, "The patient has a temperature," or "The patient has no temperature," since everyone has a temperature, abnormal or not. Edit such phrases as follows:

The patient has a fever.
or The patient is febrile.
or The patient has an elevated temperature.
or The patient has a temperature of 101.3.

The patient has no fever.
or The patient is afebrile.

Express temperature degrees with numerals except for zero.

zero degrees
48 degrees
48°

Use *minus* (not the symbol) to indicate temperatures below zero.

minus 48°C

If the temperature scale name (Celsius, Fahrenheit, Kelvin) or abbreviation (C, F, K) is not dictated, it is not necessary to insert it.

98° *or* 98 degrees

Use degree symbol (°) if available, immediately followed by abbreviation for temperature scale. If degree sign is not available, write out *degrees* (and temperature scale name, if dictated).

48°C *or* 48 degrees Celsius
98°F *or* 98 degrees Fahrenheit

Celsius
Metric-system temperature scale, designed by and named for Celsius, Swedish astronomer. Also known as *centigrade scale,* but *Celsius* is preferred term. In Celsius system, zero represents freezing point of water, 100 degrees represents boiling point at sea level. Abbreviation: C (no period). Normal human temperature on Celsius scale is 36.7.

36.7°C
or 36.7 degrees Celsius

Fahrenheit
Temperature scale designed by and named for Fahrenheit, a German-born physicist who also invented the mercury thermometer. Normal human temperature on Fahrenheit scale is 98.6.

92°F
or 92 degrees Fahrenheit

Kelvin
Temperature scale based on Celsius but not identical. Used to record extremely high and low temperatures in science. Starting point is zero, representing total absence of heat and equal to minus 273.15 degrees Celsius. To convert to Kelvin from Celsius, subtract 273.15 from Celsius temperature. Abbreviation: K (no period).

Capitalize *Kelvin* in references to the temperature scale, but lowercase *kelvin* when referring to the SI temperature unit. Abbreviation is always capitalized.

See International System of Measuring Units

tense, verb
See verbs

ter
    See personal names, nicknames, and initials

tera-
    Prefix meaning 1 trillion units of a measure. To convert to basic unit, move decimal point 12 places to the right, adding zeros as necessary.

    3.6 teratons = 3,600,000,000,000 tons

territories

Canadian territories
    See Canada

US territories
    Follow the spelling in the US Postal Service Directory of Post Offices.

    See USPS guidelines

that

conjunction
    May be omitted after a verb such as *said, stated, announced, argued,* provided its absence will not confuse the reader about the intended meaning.

    The patient said she was weak and dizzy.
    or The patient said that she was weak and dizzy.
    but The patient said today that she would exercise.
    not The patient said today she would exercise.
    (Without that, *the reader cannot determine if she said it today or she is going to exercise today.)*

introduction to essential clause
    Use *that* or *which* to introduce an essential clause referring to an inanimate object or to an animal without a name.

    The patient came into the emergency room, and she was treated for tachycardia *that had resisted conversion in her physician's office.*

She had two large wounds *that were bleeding profusely* and several small bleeders.

When *that* as a conjunction is used elsewhere in the same sentence, use *which,* not *that,* to introduce an essential clause.

It was determined that the dog which bit the child was rabid.

See clauses

that is
Latin equivalents are *i.e.* and *viz.*

See Latin abbreviations

the
Definite article. Compare *a, an.*

See articles

thousand
Quantities dictated in the form "four point two thousand" may be transcribed as 4.2 thousand or as 4200.

Thursday
See days of the week

t.i.d.
See drug terminology

tilde accent mark (~)
See accent marks

time

abbreviations
Do not abbreviate English units of time except in virgule constructions and tables. Do not use periods with such abbreviations.

The patient is 5 days old.
He will return in 3 weeks for followup.
40 mm/h

In virgule constructions (and tables), use the following abbreviations from the SI (International System of Measuring Units). Note that no periods are used.

minute   min
week   wk
month   mo
hour   h
day   d
year   y

Abbreviate Latin expressions of time, and use periods.

q.h.
q.i.d.
q.4h.

Do not confuse English abbreviations *h* and *d* (hour and day) with Latin abbreviations *h.* and *d.* (hora and die).

q.4h. *not* q.4h

hours and minutes
Use numerals, separated by a colon, to express hours and minutes, except for midnight and noon. For on-the-hour expressions, it is preferable not to add the colon and *00. See* military time *below.*

8:15 a.m.
but 8 a.m. *or* 8 o'clock in the morning, *not* 8:00 a.m., *not* 8:00 o'clock,
    not 8 a.m. o'clock, *not* 8 o'clock a.m., *not* eight o'clock

noon *not* 12 o'clock
midnight *not* 12 o'clock

military time
Identifies the day's 24 hours by numerals 1 through 24, rather than 1 a.m. through noon and 1 p.m. through midnight. Hours 1 through 12 are consistent with a.m. hours 1 through 12, while hours 13 through 24 correlate with p.m. hours 1 through 12, respectively. This form always takes four numerals, so insert the preceding or following zeros as necessary.

Do not separate hours from minutes with a colon or otherwise. Do not use *a.m.* or *p.m.*

1300 hours
0845 hours

possessive adjectives
Use *'s* or *s'*, whichever is appropriate, with units of time used as possessive adjectives.

one year's experience
two months' history
three days' time

time sequence
Give hours, minutes, seconds, tenths, hundredths in that sequence, using figures and punctuation as follows:

8:45:4.78

time span
Use hyphenated construction in a descriptive adjectival phrase expressing a time span.

one-month course
3-day period

Do not separate related time-span units by punctuation.

Labor lasted 8 hours 15 minutes.

See
a.m., AM; p.m., PM
clock referents
International System of Measuring Units
time zones
years, decades, centuries

time zones

In extended forms, capitalize only those terms that are always capitalized, e.g., Atlantic, Pacific. Note: Some references capitalize Eastern, but some do not; be consistent. Lowercase *standard time* and *daylight time.*

Daylight time is also known as daylight-saving time. Either form is correct, except that when linking the term to the name of a time zone, use *daylight time,* not *daylight-saving time.* Do not capitalize. Do not hyphenate.

Pacific daylight time

abbreviations

Use the abbreviation only when it accompanies a clock reading. Use all capitals in abbreviated forms, with no periods. Do not use commas before or after the abbreviation.

10 a.m. EST
Eastern standard time is ...

event time

The time in the zone where an event occurs determines the date (and time) of the event.

times symbol (x)
See x

titles

commas

Lowercase titles that are set off from a name by commas.

The 1994 AAMT secretary, Bonnie Monico, read the minutes.

compound forms

Use a hyphen in some compound titles, not in others. Check appropriate references for guidance.

vice president
president-elect
editor in chief
attorney at law

courtesy titles

Courtesy titles include *Mr., Mrs., Ms.,* and *Miss.* Their use is diminishing except in letter salutations. Abbreviate when they accompany a full name or surname. The use of periods following such titles (except *Miss*) continues to be prevalent, but there is a trend toward dropping them.

When a woman's preference for Ms., Miss, or Mrs. is known, use it; when it is not known, use *Ms.*

Ms. White

If a woman retains her maiden name upon marriage, use *Ms.,* not *Mrs.*

Claudia Tessier *or* Ms. Claudia Tessier *not* Mrs. Claudia Tessier

If a woman takes her husband's name, use either *Ms.* or *Mrs.,* whichever is her preference; if you don't know, use *Ms.* Avoid addressing a female patient by her husband's given name and surname because it is less specific for identification purposes; when such form is used, precede it by *Mrs.,* not *Ms.*

Rathany Aellos *or* Ms. Rathany Aellos *or* Mrs. Victor Aellos
not Ms. Victor Aellos

When referring to husband and wife together, use one of the following forms:

Lori and Tim Smith
or Tim and Lori Smith *(no courtesy titles)*

Ms. Terri Wakefield and Mr. Keith Wakefield
or Mr. Keith Wakefield and Ms. Terri Wakefield
or Mr. and Mrs. Keith Wakefield

In salutations, use a courtesy title only with the last name, not with first and last name.

Dear Ms. Wilder *not* Dear Ms. Shirley Wilder

When the salutation includes more than one person, precede each by a courtesy title, unless the same courtesy title applies to all, in which case its plural form may be used (use extended form, not abbreviation, for plural courtesy titles in salutations).

> Dear Rev. and Mrs. Jones:
> Dear Ms. Tessier and Mr. Bryon:
> Dear Doctors Gray and White:
> *or* Dear Dr. Gray and Dr. White:
> *not* Dear Drs. Gray and White:

Do not use courtesy titles when other titles, degrees, or credentials are used.

> Genny Smith, CMT
> *not*
> Ms. Genny Smith, CMT

When a courtesy title for an academic degree, e.g., *Dr.*, precedes a name, do not use the degree abbreviation after the name. Use one form or the other.

> Dr. John Wilson *or* John Wilson, MD *not* Dr. John Wilson, MD

Do not separate a courtesy title from the name it accompanies, i.e., do not allow the courtesy title to appear at the end of one line and the name on the next line.

> After a lengthy examination of the patient,
> Dr. Madison concluded ...
> *not* After a lengthy examination of the patient, Dr.
> Madison concluded ...

false titles

A person's position of employment is not necessarily a title. Avoid making formal titles out of job position names, job description designations, occupational titles, or other labels, which always take the lowercase. *See* occupational titles *below.*

> Melissa Flores, AAMT member services coordinator
> AAMT's recertification staff assistant, Ann Bianchi

formal titles

Capitalize formal titles that precede a name and are not set off by commas. A formal title denotes scope of authority or professional accomplishment so specific that it is an integral part of the person's identity.

Attorney General Janet Reno

Capitalize a formal title before a name even if it is a former, temporary, or about-to-be conferred title of the individual, provided it is not set off by commas. Do not capitalize the modifying word(s) accompanying it.

former President Bush

Abbreviate the following formal titles when used before a name.

Dr.
Gov.
Lt. Gov.
Rep.
Sen.

Lowercase formal titles not used with a name.

The surgeon general spoke at our meeting.

Lowercase formal titles that follow a name. Use commas to set off such titles.

Robert Reich, secretary of labor, is interested in the impact of electronic monitoring on employees.

Avoid constructions such as *surgeon Martin White.* Instead, insert *the* before the title.

the surgeon, Martin White

If uncertain whether a title is formal and should be capitalized, insert *the* before it and set it off by commas.

the attorney general, Janet Reno
Janet Reno, the attorney general, ...

Lowercase titles that are not formal titles, whether they precede or follow a name. *See* occupational titles *below.*

Ruth T. Gross, chief of pediatrics
Ralph Emerson, St. John's Hospital administrator
the department head, Dr. Janeway

job descriptions, job titles
   See occupational titles *below.*

military titles
   Capitalize when used as a formal title before a person's name.

   General Eisenhower

   Lowercase such titles when they stand alone.

   The general ...

   The abbreviated form is acceptable only before a person's name.
The abbreviation may be followed by a period, but it is not required.

   Gen. Bradley *or* Gen Bradley
   1st Lt. Wilder *or* 1st Lt Wilder (*at beginning of sentence:* First
        Lieutenant Wilder ...)
   Capt. Kidd *or* Capt Kidd

occupational titles
   Always lowercase occupational titles. Do not confuse them with
official titles. If not certain whether a title is occupational or official,
assume it is occupational and do not capitalize it even if it precedes the
name.

   Linda Byrne, CMT, is MTCP certification coordinator.

publication titles
   Italicize names of books and journals; if italics are not available,
underline them. Place quotation marks around names of book chapters
or journal articles.
   Capitalize major words in titles of publications and their parts. Do
not capitalize a conjunction, article, or preposition of three letters or less
(unless it is the first or last word in the title). Capitalize two-letter verbs
and both parts of dual verbs in titles.

Dorland's Illustrated Medical Dictionary
"Treating AIDS in Children" is chapter 12 in this pediatrics text.
Paris Is Burning

signature block titles
Use initial capitals for titles that follow a name in a signature block.

Ruth T. Gross, MD
Chief of Pediatrics

See Dr., Dr

TNM classification of malignant tumors
See cancer classifications

tomorrow
Replace tomorrow with the date to which it refers except in direct quotations.

D *(on May 4)*: She will return tomorrow.
T: She will return May 5.

ton
US ton, also known as a short ton, equals 2000 pounds. British ton, also known as a long ton, equals 2240 pounds. Metric ton equals 1000 kilograms (approximately 2204.62 pounds).

tonight
Do not combine with *p.m.*

8 tonight *or* 8 o'clock tonight *or* 8 p.m.
not 8 p.m. tonight

Quality is everyone's responsibility.
W. Edwards Deming

total quality management
A system of management that emphasizes continuous quality improvement. It has great potential for application to medical transcription. Abbreviation: TQM (no periods).

See
Appendix X, "Total Quality Management and Medical Transcription"
Appendix Z, "Debunking False Assumptions about Quality Management"
Appendix AA, "The Empowered Transcriptionist: A Valued Member of the Health Records Team"

town
See state, county, city, and town names and resident designations

TPAL terminology
See obstetrics terminology

TQM
Abbreviation for *total quality management.*

See total quality management

trade name, trademark
See
drug terminology
names

transcribed but not read
Sometimes transcriptionists are directed to enter this statement at the end of a transcribed report. Since the MT can verify only the first word (*transcribed*), and only the dictator can verify the second and third (*not read*), and the latter is a fact that may change later, it is not appropriate for the MT to enter the statement. In addition, not reading records is a practice MTs should not encourage. If, nevertheless, the MT is required to enter this statement, it is advisable for the MT to get the directive in writing, to document his/her objections to it, and to retain that documentation should it be necessary to defend the action in the future.

See
audit trails
authentication
dictated but not read
risk management

transcribed verbatim
See verbatim transcription

The ill and unfitting choice of words wonderfully obstructs the understanding.
Francis Bacon

transcriber
A machine used to listen to dictation for transcription purposes. Do not use *transcriber* to refer to the person who transcribes. Change to *medical transcriptionist* or *medical language specialist*.

It is a common but erroneous practice to call any transcriber a Dictaphone. Dictaphone is a corporation, and its name is trademarked. Therefore, it should be used only to refer to Dictaphone products.

transcriptionist
See medical transcriptionist

transcriptionist initials
See formats

transitional phrases
See phrases

trauma score
See scores

Tuesday
> *See* days of the week

two-letter state abbreviations
> *See*
> Appendix CC, "State Names and Abbreviations, Major Cities, and
>   State/City Resident Designations"
> state, county, city, and town names and resident designations
> USPS guidelines

type
> For most applications as an adjective, lowercase *type* and use roman
> numerals or capital letters. Check appropriate references for guidance.

> type II hyperlipoproteinemia
> type A personality

> Avoid use of *type* as a verb in reference to medical transcription. Use
> *transcribe* instead.

> The MT transcribed the report.
> *not* The MT typed the report.

type font
> Set of type of a particular size and style. The choice of type font
> influences line length, so the meaning of *line* as a unit of measure for
> transcription is useless unless the length of it (number of characters in
> a line, not number of inches) is specified.

> *See* line count

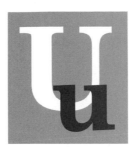

u.d.
   See drug terminology

umlaut accent mark (¨)
   See accent marks

unattached modifier
   See dangling modifiers

under
   Do not use to mean *less than.* If this meaning is intended, use *less than* instead.

   D: She weighed under 80 pounds.
   T: She weighed less than 80 pounds.

underlining
   Avoid as much as possible because it reduces readability. Use regular type instead, or if type must be distinguished from regular type, use italics or boldface. If underlining must be used, underline the full phrase, including spaces and punctuation, except final punctuation.

United States
   Abbreviate (*US* or *U.S.*) only when used as a modifier.

   She came to the United States in 1983.

She became a US citizen in 1989.

units of measure

metric system

System of weights and measures based upon the meter. Units are increased by multiples of 10, decreased by divisors of 10. Prefixes are added to denote fractional or multiple units.

deci-	one-tenth
centi-	one-hundredth
milli-	one-thousandth
micro-	one-millionth
nano-	one-billionth
pico-	one-trillionth
deka-	10 units
hecto-	100 units
kilo-	1000 units
mega-	one million units
giga-	one billion units
tera-	one trillion units

Note: Individual, commonly used metric units of measure are listed alphabetically in this text.

Use abbreviations when a numeric quantity precedes the metric unit of measure; never use periods and never add *s* to plural form. Write out the unit of measure if the quantity is written out.

14 mg *not* 14 milligrams *not* 14 mg. *not* 14 mgs *not* 14 mgs.
10 mm/h

Do not capitalize most metric units of measure or their abbreviations. Learn the obvious exceptions, and consult appropriate references for guidance.

centimeter	cm
hertz	Hz
decibel	dB
liter	L (*preferred to* l)

Use the decimal form with metric measurements even when dictated as a fraction.

4.5 mm *not* 4 ½ mm

nonmetric units of measure
Spell out common nonmetric units of measure (*pound, ounce, inch, foot, yards, mile,* etc.) to express depth, distance, height, length, weight, and width, except in tables. Do not use an apostrophe or quotation marks to indicate *feet* or *inches,* respectively (except in tables).

4 pounds
5 ounces
14 inches
5 feet
5 feet 3 inches *not* 5' 3" *not* 5 ft. 3 in.

Do not abbreviate most nonmetric units of measure, except in tables. Use the same abbreviation for both singular and plural forms; do not add *s.*

1 in., 5 in.

Do not use a comma or other punctuation between units of the same dimension.

The infant weighed 5 pounds 3 ounces.
He is 5 feet 4 inches tall.

hyphens
Use a hyphen to join a number and a unit of measure when they are used as an adjective preceding a noun.

4.5-mm incision
5-inch wound

numerals
Do not allow a numeral to end one line of type and its accompanying unit of measure (abbreviated or not) to begin the next line. Use a required space or coded space or nonbreaking space between them to assure that the numerals move to the next line along with the abbreviation.

....5 cm
not
....5
cm

series
    Do not repeat units of measure in a related series.

    4 x 5 cm
    140, 135, and 58 cc

verb-subject agreement
    Units of measure are collective singular nouns and take singular verbs.

    Twenty milliequivalents of KCl was given.

    See
    abbreviations
    decimals, decimal units
    drug terminology
    exponents
    fractions
    International System of Measuring Units
    numbers
    solutions
    time

units of time
    See
    International System of Measuring Units
    time

universal present
    See verbs

unnecessary verbs
    See verbs

unparallel series
    See series

uppercase, uppercased
One word, no hyphen.

urinalysis
Term evolved from *urine analysis,* which is now archaic. Edit to *urinalysis.* Use abbreviation *UA* only if dictated.

D: Urine analysis showed ...
T: Urinalysis showed ...

US, U.S.
Abbreviations for *United States.* Use only as an adjective and only if dictated. Use capital letters, with or without periods.

USP system
United States Pharmacopeia system for sizing sutures.

See suture sizes

USPS guidelines
USPS is abbreviation for US Postal Service.

This section was adapted from *A Guide to Business Mail Preparation,* a copy of which is available from your US Post Office if you would like additional directions regarding proper addressing of business mail.

definitions
Domestic mail: Mail transmitted within, among, and between the United States; its territories and possessions; the areas comprising the former Canal Zone; Army/Air Force (APO) and Navy (FPO) post offices; and mail for delivery to the United Nations, New York. The term "territories and possessions" includes:

Baker Island
Canton Island
Caroline Islands
Enderbury Island
Guam
Howland Island
Jarvis Island

Johnston Island
Kingman Reef
Manua Island
Marshall Islands, Republic of the
Midway Islands
Navassa Island
Northern Mariana Islands, Commonwealth of
    the Palau
Puerto Rico, Commonwealth of
Saint Croix Island
Saint John Island
Saint Thomas Island
Samoa (American)
Sand Island
Swain's Island
Trust Territory of the Pacific
Virgin Islands (U.S.)
Wake Island

International mail: Mail addressed to or received from foreign countries

address guidelines

To facilitate automated handling of mail, US Postal Service guidelines call for envelopes to be addressed in all capitals, without use of punctuation marks. The use of ZIP codes is recommended on all mail to enable the Postal Service to achieve greater reliability and efficiency in dispatch and delivery.

ZIP is the abbreviation for *Zone Improvement Program*. ZIP codes are five- or nine-digit codes (ZIP plus four). Use of the nine-digit ZIP code is preferred over the five-digit ZIP code; use a hyphen or en dash between the first five and last four digits. Use ZIP-plus-four codes in return addresses, as well.

ZIP code abbreviations are USPS two-letter abbreviations for US states, territories, and possessions. Capitalize the two letters and place a single space but no comma between the ZIP code abbreviation and the ZIP code in a mailing address.

USPS preferred address formats (domestic mail):

> SUSAN B SMITH
> 876 LAKE ST
> ST LOUIS MO 63135-2134

SUSAN B SMITH
876 LAKE ST STE M
ST LOUIS MO 63135-2134

SUSAN B SMITH
876 LAKE ST APT 18
ST LOUIS MO 63135-2134

SUSAN B SMITH
PO BOX 6187
DALLAS TX 75201

SUSAN B SMITH
RR 2 BOX 89
MODESTO CA 95357

SUSAN SMITH CMT
MEDICAL TRANSCRIPTION DEPT
ST ANNE HOSPITAL
Mail will be delivered here .. 1111 CENTRAL ST
ST LOUIS MO 63135-2134

TRANSMED INC
Attention note here .... ATTN SUSAN SMITH
1608 WILSON ST
NEW YORK NY 10001-0200

Specific directions here .... PERSONAL AND CONFIDENTIAL TO
SUSAN SMITH
TRANSMED INC
1608 WILSON ST
NEW YORK NY 10001-0200

TRANSMED INC
1608 WILSON ST
Mail will be delivered here .. PO BOX 200 GRAND STATION
NEW YORK NY 10001-0200

TRANSMED INC
PO BOX 200 GRAND STATION
Mail will be delivered here .. 1608 WILSON STREET
NEW YORK NY 10001-0200

For mail on which space or other factors make positioning of the ZIP code following the city impractical, the ZIP code may be placed at the bottom line of the address, provided it is immediately beneath the city and state and no characters or digits precede or follow it.

MR JAMES SMITH
1861 MAIN ST
BATON ROUGE LA
70805-5868

Mail to Canada: Mail addressed to Canada may use either of the following formats when the postal delivery zone number is included in the address:

MRS JANE SMITH
2121 LAKE ST
OTTAWA ON K1A OB1
CANADA

MRS JANE SMITH
2121 LAKE ST
OTTAWA ON CANADA
K1A OB1

International mail: Mail addressed to a foreign country should include the country name printed in capital letters (no abbreviations) as the only information on the bottom line.

MR JAMES SMITH
117 CLINTON ST
LONDON WIP6HQ
ENGLAND

See
addresses
Appendix CC, "State Names and Abbreviations, Major Cities, and
    State/City Resident Designations"
state, county, city, and town names and resident designations

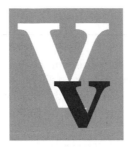

v
> *See*
> verbs
> versus

VA
> *See*
> Veterans Administration
> visual acuity

value added
> *See* Appendix BB, "'Value Added' Defined"

> ### *Value has been defined as*
> ### *the ability to command the price.*
> Louis Dembitz Brandeis

van, von
> *See* personal names, nicknames, and initials

verb-subject agreement

A verb must agree in number with the noun that serves as its subject. Use a singular verb with a singular subject, a plural verb with a plural subject.

The *abdomen is* soft and nontender.
The *lungs are* clear.

The verb must agree with its subject even when the two are not in proximity. Be especially careful when another noun intervenes.

The *findings* on tomography *were* normal.

Take care to accurately identify the subject; inaccurate identification can lead to errors in the number of the verb.

He is one of those patients who demand constant reassurance. (The subject of *demand* is *who,* referring to *patients,* not to *he.*)

What surprised me was the symptoms were not typical. (The subject is *what surprised me,* not *the symptoms,* so *was* is the appropriate verb.)

Collective nouns may be singular or plural and take the matching verb.

See
amount of
average of
either...or, neither...nor
everyone, every one
money
nouns
number of
units of measure
verbs

***Those who write as they speak, even though
they speak well, write badly.***
Comte de Buffon

verbatim transcription

Most dictation cannot be transcribed verbatim if it is to be complete, comprehensible, and consistent, since few people speak in a manner that allows conversion into printed form without at least minor editing.

Nevertheless, some medical transcriptionists are required to transcribe some or all reports verbatim. Unless the dictation is perfect (which is unlikely), the MT should retain some evidence of the directive, preferably entering the statement "transcribed verbatim" at the end of the report, in order to defend the transcript in the future if necessary.

AAMT has prepared a tape titled *More to It Than Meets the Ear,* with excerpts of challenging dictation, demonstrating the reality of medical transcription. For price information, contact AAMT at 800-982-2182 or 209-551-0883, or fax 209-551-9317.

See
audit trails
editing
risk management

verbs

Verbs express action or being. The abbreviation *v* is used in this book to indicate verb forms. Verbs have mood, person and number, tense, and voice.

mood

The indicative mood makes factual statements and is most common.

The patient returned on schedule for a followup visit.

The imperative mood makes requests or demands.

Come here now.

The subjunctive mood expresses doubt, wishes, regrets, or conditions contrary to fact. It is the most difficult and most formal mood and usually relates to the past or present, not the future.

indicative	He is a singer.
imperative	Clean up your room.
subjunctive	If she were my patient, I would proceed with surgery.

person and number

Person expresses the entity (first, second, or third) that is acting or being. *Number* expresses whether the person is singular or plural.

first person singular	I
second person singular	you *(one only)*
third person singular	he *or* she
first person plural	we
second person plural	you *(more than one)*
third person plural	they

> ### There's no present. There's only the immediate future and the recent past.
> George Carlin

tense

Use verb tense to communicate the appropriate time of the action or being: past, present, future, past perfect, perfect, and future perfect. Maintain uniformity of tense, but keep in mind that tense may vary within a single report or even a single paragraph, depending on the time being referenced.

D: The abdomen is soft. There was a scar in the lower right quadrant.
T: The abdomen is soft. There is a scar in the lower right quadrant.

Tenses may appropriately vary within a single paragraph and certainly within a report.

She was admitted from the emergency room at 8:30 p.m. She is afebrile at present. She will be given IV antibiotics, nevertheless.

historic present: Uses the present tense to relate past events in a more immediate manner. In dictation, it is common to use the historic tense to describe patient information or treatment in the present rather than in the past. If this is done, be consistent. The historic present is not the same as the *universal present* (see below).

The *patient says she has* pain over the right abdomen.
Upon examination, *there is* rebound tenderness.

universal present: Uses the present tense to state something is universally true or that was believed to be true at the time. The universal present is not the same as the *historic present* (see above).

Traditional treatment modalities were used because *they are* so effective.

voice
In the active voice, the subject is the doer. In the passive voice, the subject is done unto. Most communication guidelines urge use of the active voice except when it is more important to emphasize what was acted on and that it was acted on.
In medical transcription, the active voice is more common in reporting observations, e.g., in history and physical exam reports, while the passive voice is more common in describing healthcare providers' actions, e.g., hospital treatment and surgery.

The abdomen is soft, nontender.
The patient was given intravenous aminophylline.
The incision was made over the symphysis pubis.

Do not recast most dictation to change the voice except for those sentences which are especially awkward. The most common instance when it is necessary to change voice is in dictation by physicians for whom English is a second language, especially if their English sentence structure reflects that of their native tongue rather than of English.

D: The medication by him is taken irregularly.
T: He takes the medication irregularly.

linking verbs
Verbs that link the subject of a sentence to an adjective or other complement. Examples include *act, appear, feel, look, be, remain, become, get, grow, seem, smell, sound,* and *taste.* Such verbs are followed by adjectives, not adverbs, because the subject, not the verb, is being described.

He says the food tastes bad.
not He says the food tastes badly.

split verbs

A split verb is one in which a word (usually an adverb) has been inserted between its two parts. Splitting infinitives or other forms of verbs used to be considered a grave grammatical sin. Traditionalists still hold to this view, but pragmatists recognize that such splits are appropriate if they enhance meaning (or at least do not obstruct it). Transcribe split verbs as dictated provided they do not obstruct the meaning.

The test was intended *to* definitively *determine* ...
He *will* routinely *return* for followup.

> *...when I split an infinitive, God dammit,*
> *I split it so it will stay split.*
> Raymond Chandler

unnecessary verbs

In comparisons such as the following, the second verb is understood.

The larger incision healed faster than the smaller one.

If the second verb is dictated or added, be sure to place it at the end.

The larger incision healed faster than the smaller one did.
not
The larger incision healed faster than did the smaller one.

See verb-subject agreement

Veress needle

The correct spelling is *Veress* although many references continue to use the incorrect spelling *Verres*.

versus

Abbreviation: v or vs (lowercased, no period) or v., vs. (lowercased, period). Do not abbreviate in most instances (exception: referencing a court case).

Roe v Wade

vertebra

Expressed by a capital C, L, T, or S to indicate the region (cervical, lumbar, thoracic, or sacral), followed by an arabic numeral placed on-line (do not subscript or superscript). D for *dorsal* is sometimes substituted for T (thoracic). Do not use a hyphen between the letter and the number of a specific vertebra. Do not subscript or superscript the numerals. Plural: vertebrae.

S1 *not* S-1
T2 *or* D2

It is preferable to repeat the letter before each numbered vertebra.

C5 and C6 *not* C5 and 6

intervertebral disk space
Use a hyphen to express the space between two vertebrae (the intervertebral space).

S1-S2
L5-S1

vertical series
See
lists
outlines
series

Veterans Administration

Veterans is used as a noun-adjective not as a possessive, so no apostrophe. Abbreviation: *VA* (no periods).

Veterans Administration Hospital

vice

Do not hyphenate in titles.

vice president
vice admiral

virgule (/)

The virgule, also known as *diagonal, slash,* or *solidus,* is used for a variety of purposes.

accent mark
    See accent marks

and / or
    Use a virgule to refer equally to the entity on each side of the virgule or to both together, for example when gender is not specified and does not matter. *See* duality *below.*

his/her

in dates
    Virgules may be used to separate numerals representing the month, day, and year in tables and figures. This form is also used for admission and discharge dates when giving patient demographic data. Do not use hyphens instead of virgules. Do not use virgules in dates in textual matter, i.e., within reports; write out dates instead.

Admission: 4/4/94 *not* 4-4-94
Discharge: 4/9/94 *not* 4-9-94

The patient was seen on April 4, 1994.
not The patient was seen on 4/4/94.

duality
    Use a virgule to imply duality, i.e., that the entity on each side of the virgule is the same as the other. When the two entities are not the same; use another punctuation mark, e.g., the hyphen. *See* and/or *above.*

physician/patient (one person; physician as patient)
physician-patient relationship (two people)

employer-employee relationship
not employer/employee relationship

fractions
Use a virgule to separate the numerator from the denominator in fractions.

4/5
2/3
1/2

over
Use a virgule to express *over* in expressions such as the following.

blood pressure 160/100
grade 1/4 murmur

per
To express *per* with a virgule, there must be at least one specific numeric quantity, and the element immediately on each side of the virgule must be either a specific numeric quantity or a unit of measurement.

Do not use a virgule if the unit of measure does not have an acceptable abbreviated form, when a prepositional phrase intervenes between the elements between *per,* or in nontechnical phrases.

Sed rate: 52 mm/h
120 beats per minute *not* 120 beats/min

She takes 5 mg of Valium per day.
not She takes 5 mg of Valium/day.

She weighs in three days per week.
not She weighs in 3 d/w.

Do not use more than one virgule per expression.

4 ml/kg per minute *not* 4 ml/kg/min

visual acuity
Express with arabic numerals separated by a virgule.

Visual acuity: 20/200 corrected to 20/40.

See
dates
fractions

virus names

Viruses have both vernacular (common) and official names. Do not capitalize most common or vernacular virus names, except for eponyms associated with them.

herpesvirus
herpes simplex virus
Epstein-Barr virus

Capitalize official (family, subfamily) names. The endings *-idae* and *-inae* indicate such terms.

Parvoviridae (family)
Oncovirinae (subfamily)

The ending *-virus* usually indicates an official term but sometimes indicates a vernacular term. The vernacular usage usually makes *virus* a separate word, but not always.

Rotavirus (family)
parvovirus (vernacular)
rubella virus (vernacular)

When two or more forms are acceptable, choose one and use it consistently.

papovavirus *or* PaPoVa virus

Some virus names derive from combinations of words, as a kind of acronym. Some that were originally capitalized are now preferred lowercased.

echovirus (enteric cytopathic human orphan virus; previously expressed as ECHOvirus)

Use arabic numerals in most series designations of virus, but use roman numerals in the HTLV series.

LAV-1 (lymphadenopathy-associated virus type 1)
HTLV-II (human T-cell lymphotropic virus type II)

visual acuity
Express with arabic numerals separated by a virgule. Abbreviation: VA (no periods).

His visual acuity of 20/200 is corrected to 20/40.

vitamins
See drug terminology

viz.
See Latin abbreviations

volume
Use a lowercased x and numerals in expressions of volume.

2 x 3 x 4 m^3

Use liters to show liquid or gas volume, cubic meters to show solid volumes.

3 L
4 m^3

See International System of Measuring Units

von, van
See personal names, nicknames, and initials

vs, vs.
See versus

vulgarities
See obscenities, profanities, vulgarities

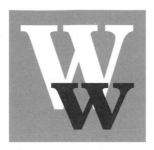

wbc, WBC
    See blood counts

Wednesday
    See days of the week

weight
    Express with numerals. Spell out *pounds* and *ounces* except in tables. Do not separate the pounds expression from the ounces expression by *and,* a comma, or other punctuation when they are a unit.

    The infant weighed 4 pounds 5 ounces. (*not* 4 lb. 5 oz., *not* 4 pounds, 5 ounces)

    Use abbreviations for metric units of weight.

    5 g
    24 kg

    See numbers

west, western, West, Western
    See north, south, east, west

whether or not

Drop *or not* when *whether* means *if,* which implies an alternative. Retain *or not* when the intended meaning is *regardless.* Determine whether to retain *or not* by testing the sentence without it.

Some use *or not* whether or not it is needed.
We will determine whether (*if*) he needs surgery after the lab
results are available.

which, that

See clauses *to determine when to use* which *or* that.

white

See sociocultural designations

white blood cells, white blood count

See blood counts

who, whom

Use to refer to human beings. Use *who* as the subject of a sentence or clause. Use *whom* as the object of a verb or preposition.

See clauses

who's, whose

who's
Contraction for *who is.*

Who's questioning my diagnosis?

whose
Possessive form of *who.*

Whose idea was it to admit this patient?

width
Express with numerals.

See numbers

will, shall
Usage distinctions between *will* and *shall* are lessening except in legal documents. Transcribe as dictated.

winter
See seasons

woman, women
See age referents

word division
Avoiding end-of-line word division facilitates both communication and transcription: the reader of the document does not lose the flow of reading and meaning, and the medical transcriptionist does not have to hesitate or stop to determine correct word division.

If you choose to use end-of-line word division, follow the rules for medical- and English-word division. Consult appropriate medical or English references for guidance with specific terms.

Medical words are generally divided between word parts. It is preferable to divide after a prefix or before a suffix rather than within the root word.

esophago-gastro-duodenoscopy
hyper-lipo-proteinemia
hyper-tensive
radio-immuno-assay
ultra-sound

In general, English words are divided between syllables and according to pronunciation. This is the system in most US dictionaries.

Do not divide a word in a manner that will not leave at least three characters (including the hyphen) on the first line and at least three characters (including a punctuation mark, if any) on the next line.

incorrect: e-radicate
            a-cetic

Do not divide words of one syllable. Remember that when *-ed* is added to some words, they remain one syllable and so must not be divided.

bought
caught
crossed

Divide words of two or more syllables between syllables.

fur-ther
tran-scrip-tion-ist

Divide between two adjacent vowels within a word.

tubo-ovarian
deteri-oration

Do not divide words of five or fewer letters.

bowel
cocci
into
major
prior
upper

Do not divide words of two syllables when one of the syllables is a single vowel.

abides
events

Do not divide words when the result will be a confusing syllable on either line of the transcript.

fat-test

Do not divide words that have a different meaning when divided.

re-create

Avoid dividing a word before a single-vowel syllable unless the vowel is the first syllable of a word root or suffix, e.g., *-able* or *-ible*. When the *a* or *i* in *-able* or *-ible* is pronounced with the letter(s) preceding it, divide the word after the *a* or *i*.

thera-pist, *not* ther-apist
remark-able
capa-ble
palpa-ble

When the final consonant of a verb is doubled to form the past tense or the participle, the second consonant is a part of the letters following it.

admit-ting
commit-ted

A two-letter syllable may end a line (the hyphen is the required third character), but avoid carrying a two-letter word-ending to the next line.

.................The patient was admitted

..............................We suggested that ...

not
.....................We suggested that

Divide compound words containing hyphens at the existing hyphen.

well-nourished
not well-nour-ished

Divide words compounded of other words and written as one word at natural breaks.

bedtime: bed-time
eyeglasses: eye-glasses
eyegrounds: eye-grounds

Divide a word with a prefix after the prefix, not at another point.

extra-curricular
retro-active

Divide most words ending in *ing* just before the *ing*.

experienc-ing

Avoid dividing proper names. If this cannot be avoided, break between words, not within them.

.....................................Presbyterian
Hospital
not
.....................................Presby-
terian Hospital

In particular, avoid dividing a person's name. If this cannot be avoided, make the break between the middle initial and last name or between the first and last names if there is no middle initial.

.....................................John F.
Kennedy
not
.....................................John
F. Kennedy

Do not separate a title from a proper name.

....Dr. Dirckx
not
....Dr.
Dirckx

....John Dirckx, MD
not
....John Dirckx,
MD

Do not divide abbreviations or acronyms.

wbc's

MAST
AHIMA

Do not divide numbers.

3400
45,587

Do not separate a numeric value from its accompanying abbreviation
or unit of measure.

....51.9 kg
not
.....................................51.90
kg

Divide dates between the day and the year, not between the month
and the day.

...............................February 17,
1994
not
...............................February
17, 1994

Do not divide words at the end of more than two consecutive lines.

Do not divide the word at the end of the last line of a paragraph or at
the end of the last line on a page.

See syllables

World War I, World War II
Capitalize the words and use roman numerals. Abbreviations are
WWI and *WWII*.

would, should
See should, would

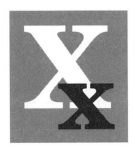

x

Use a lowercased *x* in expressions of area, volume, and magnification.

3 x 4-mm lesion
4 x 4 gauze

Use a lowercased *x* as a multiplication symbol.

42 x 38

See International System of Measuring Units

x-ray

Refers both to the radiologic process and to the radiation particles. Whether used as a noun, verb, or adjective, lowercase and hyphenate as noted.

His x-ray was not in the jacket. (n)
He was x-rayed yesterday. (v)
His x-ray films have been lost. (adj)

X rays: Their moral is this—that a right way of looking at things will see through almost anything.
Samuel Butler

Capitalize x-ray only when it is the first word in a sentence.

X-ray films showed ...

Avoid using the prefix *re-* with x-ray. Edit instead.

x-ray again
preferred to re-x-ray
not rex-ray

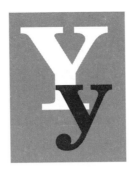

yard

Equal to three feet. Metric equivalent: approximately 0.91 meter. To convert to meters, multiply by 0.91.

Do not use abbreviation (*yd.*) except in tables. Do not use a comma or other punctuation between units of the same dimension. Express with numerals.

3 yards 2 feet 10 inches

See numbers

years, decades, centuries

years

Use numerals to express specific years. When a single year is referred to without the century, precede it by an apostrophe.

1990
'94

decades

Express with numerals except in special circumstances. Add *s* (without an apostrophe) to form the numeric plural. Use a preceding apostrophe in shortened numeric expressions relating to decades of the century ('90s), but omit the preceding apostrophe in expressions relating to decades of age (80s). Spell out and capitalize special references for decades.

the 1970s
the mid-1980s

He grew up in the '50s.
He is in his 50s.
but the Roaring Twenties, the Gay Nineties

centuries

Lowercase *century.* Spell out and lowercase century numbers *first* through *ninth;* use numerals for 10th and higher. Use a hyphen in the adjectival form.

third century
12th century
20th-century music

For proper names, use form preferred by organization.

Twentieth Century Fund
20th Century Fox

at beginning of sentence

Spell out years, decades, or centuries at the beginning of a sentence, or recast the sentence.

D: 1992 was a catastrophic year for his health.
T: The year 1992 was catastrophic for his health.

See
ages
dates
numbers

yesterday

Replace *yesterday* with the date to which it refers except in direct quotations.

D (on May 4): I saw the patient yesterday.
T: I saw the patient on May 3.

See dates

youth

See age referents

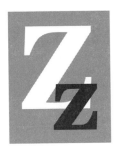

ZIP codes and ZIP code abbreviations
See
Appendix CC, "State Names and Abbreviations, Major Cities, and
    State/City Resident Designations"
state, county, city, and town names and resident designations
USPS Guidelines

...I guess the old alphabet
ISN'T enough!
NOW the letters he uses are something to see!
Most people still stop at Z...
but not He!
Dr. Seuss

The AAMT Book of Style for Medical Transcription

APPENDICES

Appendices

Appendix A, "Sample Reports" 387

Appendix B, "The Mark of Zorro," by Robert L. Love 395

Appendix C, "When Did 'CMT' Become 'MD'?" by Robert L. Love 399

Appendix D, "What's Wrong With This Picture?"
by Claudia Tessier, CAE, CMT, RRA 401

Appendix E, "AAMT Position Paper: Providers' Signatures" 409

Appendix F, "AAMT Explores Quality and Quantity Issues" 411

Appendix G, "Can You Keep a Secret?" by Pat Forbis, CMT 415

Appendix H, "Healthcare Reform and Confidentiality,"
by Kathleen Frawley, JD, RRA 419

Appendix I, "Electronic Monitoring: Outquotes and Thoughts,"
by Claudia Tessier, CAE, CMT, RRA 423

Appendix J, "Straight from the Source's Mouth,"
by Claudia Tessier, CAE, CMT, RRA 427

Appendix K, "Errors, Omissions, and the MT," by Robert L. Love 429

Appendix L, "Medical Transcription as Communication,"
by Claudia Tessier, CAE, CMT, RRA 433

Appendix M, "MTs: Partners in Medical Communication," 437

Appendix N, "The Myth of Medical Transcription,"
by Pat Forbis, CMT 443

Appendix O, "AAMT Model Job Description:
Medical Transcriptionist" 447

Appendix P, "Customizing Productivity Standards,"
by Carolyn Wilkinson, CMT 451

Appendix Q, "How Much Wood Should a Woodchuck
(or a Medical Transcriptionist) Chuck?" by Pat Forbis, CMT 457

Appendix R, "The Q-P Zone," by Terri Wakefield, CMT 461

Appendix S, "They're Asking the Wrong Questions,"
by Claudia Tessier, CAE, CMT, RRA 465

Appendix T, "Transcription by the Pound," by Pat Forbis, CMT 469

Appendix U, "AAMT Position Paper: Quality Assurance
Guidelines" 473

Appendix V, "Quality Assurance: Key to Cost Containment
in Medical Transcription," by Stella Olson, CMT 477

Appendix W, "The Quality of Patient Care Documentation,"
by Claudia Tessier, CAE, CMT, RRA 481

Appendix X, "Total Quality Management and Medical
Transcription," by Claudia Tessier, CAE, CMT, RRA 489

Appendix Y, "Medical Language," by John H. Dirckx, MD 493

Appendix Z, "Debunking False Assumptions about Quality
Management," by Claudia Tessier, CAE, CMT, RRA 497

Appendix AA, "The Empowered Transcriptionist:
A Valued Member of the Health Records Team,"
by Claire R. Jacobsen, CMT 501

Appendix BB, "'Value Added' Defined," by Pat Forbis, CMT 505

Appendix CC, "State Names and Abbreviations, Major Cities,
and State/City Resident Designations" 509

Appendix A

Sample Reports

SAMPLE REPORT – CLINIC NOTE

The patient is being seen today in followup for a bad cough, sinus congestion, and nasal discharge, worse since his last visit. He also complains of a sore on the bottom of his right foot, and he has a bulge in the left groin.

PHYSICAL EXAM
HEENT shows posterior pharyngeal drainage. The neck is supple, with tender adenopathy. TMs are clear. Lungs have some forced expiratory rhonchi. Examination of the bottom of the right foot shows a corn; I pared away some of the overlying callus. Valsalva maneuver shows a prominent left inguinal hernia; testicular exam is normal.

IMPRESSION
1. Sinusitis.
2. Corn, right foot.
3. Left inguinal hernia.

PLAN
We put him on amoxicillin 250 mg t.i.d. x 10 days. Advised him to pare the corn and use a Dr. Scholl's foot pad. We will refer him to a general surgeon regarding the left inguinal hernia. Return in two weeks if sinusitis is not improved.

NOTE: In order to conserve space in the chart, some physician offices, clinics, and other healthcare facilities format their progress notes by using section headings followed by colons, with findings beginning on the same line.

SAMPLE REPORT – SOAP NOTE

SUBJECTIVE
Jennifer is brought in for a 6-month checkup. She is doing very well. She is seeing Dr. Green for evaluation of her feet. He gave her a clean bill of health. She is on breast milk as well as cereal.

OBJECTIVE
HEENT exam is normal. Lungs are clear. Cardiac examination is within normal limits. Musculoskeletal exam is normal. Abdomen is benign. Genitalia are normal.

ASSESSMENT
Normal exam.

PLAN
Continue breast-feeding; no dietary modifications are necessary. DPT and HIB will be given.

NOTE: The SOAP format may also be used in history and physical reports. When used in clinic notes and progress notes, headings for the SOAP format may also be simplified as follows:

S:
O:
A:
P:

SAMPLE REPORT – HISTORY AND PHYSICAL

CHIEF COMPLAINT
Status post motor vehicle accident.

HISTORY OF PRESENT ILLNESS
The patient is a 17-year-old white male who is status post a high-speed motor vehicle accident in which he was ejected from the vehicle. He denies loss of consciousness, although the EMT people report that he did have loss of consciousness. The patient was stable en route. Upon arrival, he complained of headache.

PAST MEDICAL HISTORY
Medical: None. Surgical: None.

REVIEW OF SYSTEMS
CARDIAC: No history.
PULMONARY: Some morning cough. (Patient is a smoker.)

MEDICATIONS
None.

ALLERGIES
No known drug allergies.

PHYSICAL EXAMINATION
VITAL SIGNS: Blood pressure 120/80, pulse 82, respirations 20, temperature 36.8°.
HEENT: Contusion over right occiput. Tympanic membranes benign.
NECK: Nontender.
CHEST: Atraumatic, nontender.
LUNGS: Clear to auscultation and percussion.
ABDOMEN: Flat, soft, and nontender.
BACK: Atraumatic, nontender.
PELVIS: Stable.
EXTREMITIES: Contusion over right forearm. No underlying bone deformity or crepitus.
RECTAL: Normal sphincter tone; guaiac negative.
NEUROLOGIC: Glasgow coma scale 15. Pupils equal, round, reactive to light. Patient moves all four extremities without focal deficit.

LABORATORY DATA
Serial hematocrits 44.5, 42.4, and 40.4. White blood count 6.3. Ethanol: None.

(continued)

Page 2

Amylase 66. Urinalysis normal. PT 12.6, PTT 29. Chem-7 panel within normal limits.

X-rays of cervical spine and lumbosacral spine within normal limits. X-rays of pelvis and chest within normal limits.

ASSESSMENT
1. Closed head injury.
2. Rule out intra-abdominal injury.

PLAN
The patient will be admitted to the trauma surgery service for continued evaluation and treatment for closed head injury as well as possible intra-abdominal injury.

SAMPLE REPORT – CONSULTATION

REASON FOR CONSULTATION

This 92-year-old female states that last night she had a transient episode of slurred speech and numbness of her left cheek for a few hours. However, the chart indicates that she had recurrent TIAs three times yesterday, each lasting about five minutes, with facial drooping and some mental confusion. She had also complained of blurred vision for several days. She was brought to the emergency room last night, where she was noted to have a left carotid bruit and was felt to have recurrent TIAs.

The patient is on Lanoxin, amoxicillin, Hydergine, Cardizem, Lasix, Micro-K, and a salt-free diet. She does not smoke or drink alcohol.

Admission CT scan of the head showed a densely calcified mass lesion of the sphenoid bone, probably representing the benign osteochondroma seen on previous studies. CBC was normal, aside from a hemoglobin of 11.2. ECG showed atrial fibrillation. BUN was 22, creatinine normal, CPK normal, glucose normal, electrolytes normal.

PHYSICAL EXAMINATION

On examination, the patient is noted to be alert and fully oriented. She has some impairment of recent memory. She is not dysphasic, nor is she apraxic. Speech is normal and clear. The head is noted to be normocephalic. Neck is supple. Carotid pulses are full bilaterally, with left carotid bruit. Neurologic exam shows cranial nerve function II through XII to be intact, save for some slight flattening of the left nasolabial fold. Motor examination shows no drift of the outstretched arms. There is no tremor or past-pointing. Finger-to-nose and heel-to-shin performed well bilaterally. Motor showed intact neuromuscular tone, strength, and coordination in all limbs. Reflexes 1+ and symmetrical, with bilateral plantar flexion, absent jaw jerk, no snout. Sensory exam is intact to pinprick, touch, vibration, position, temperature, and graphesthesia.

IMPRESSION

Neurological examination is normal, aside from mild impairment of recent memory, slight flattening of the left nasolabial fold, and left carotid bruit. She also has atrial fibrillation, apparently chronic. In view of her age and the fact that she is in chronic atrial fibrillation, I would suspect that she most likely has had embolic phenomena as the cause of her TIAs.

(continued)

Page 2

RECOMMENDATIONS

I would recommend conservative management with antiplatelet agents unless a near-occlusion of the carotid arteries is demonstrated, in which case you might consider it best to do an angiography and consider endarterectomy. In view of her age, I would be reluctant to recommend Coumadin anticoagulation. I will be happy to follow the patient with you.

SAMPLE REPORT – OPERATION

PREOPERATIVE DIAGNOSES
1. Right spontaneous pneumothorax secondary to barometric trauma.
2. Respiratory failure.
3. Pneumonia with sepsis.

POSTOPERATIVE DIAGNOSES
1. Right spontaneous pneumothorax secondary to barometric trauma.
2. Respiratory failure.
3. Pneumonia with sepsis.

NAME OF OPERATION
Right chest tube insertion.

INDICATIONS
Spontaneous right pneumothorax secondary to barometric trauma from increased
PEEP. An early morning chest x-ray showed approximately 30% pneumothorax on
the right.

INFORMED CONSENT
Not obtained. This patient is obtunded, intubated, and septic. This is an emergent
procedure with two-physician emergency consent signed and on the chart.

PROCEDURE
The patient's right chest was prepped and draped in sterile fashion. The site of
insertion was anesthetized with 1% Xylocaine, and an incision was made. Blunt
dissection was carried out two intercostal spaces above the initial incision site. The
chest wall was opened, and a 32-French chest tube was placed into the thoracic
cavity after examination with the finger, making sure that the thoracic cavity had
been entered correctly. The chest tube was placed on wall suction and subsequently
sutured in place with 0 silk.

A postoperative chest x-ray is pending at this time. The patient tolerated the
procedure well and was taken to the recovery room in stable condition.

ESTIMATED BLOOD LOSS
10 cc.

COMPLICATIONS
None.

SAMPLE REPORT - DISCHARGE SUMMARY

ADMITTING DIAGNOSES
1. Second-degree heart block with 2:1 conduction.
2. Right bundle branch block.
3. Left anterior fascicular block.
4. Adult-onset diabetes.

HISTORY OF PRESENT ILLNESS
The patient is a 69-year-old white female who has been followed in my clinic for adult-onset diabetes. She is known to have a right bundle branch block and left anterior fascicular block on previous EKG. She presented to my office complaining of increased lethargy over the preceding week.

PHYSICAL EXAMINATION
Physical exam demonstrated bradycardia with pulse in the 40s. EKG revealed second-degree heart block with 2:1 conduction and a ventricular rate in the 40s. The patient denied any light-headedness, syncope, chest pain, shortness of breath, palpitations, history of myocardial infarction, or rhythm disturbance.

HOSPITAL COURSE
The patient was admitted directly to the hospital and admitted to a monitored floor. MI was ruled out, and cardiology consult was obtained. At that time, it was felt that the patient was in need of a permanent pacemaker. She underwent dual-chamber pacemaker insertion on the following day without complications. She has done well postoperatively, without any symptoms, and has remained in normal sinus rhythm with pacer capturing throughout observation. She is presently without complaints except for some nasal congestion and tenderness over the pacer insertion site. However, there is no erythema or discharge at the operative site. The patient is clinically stable for discharge.

DISCHARGE MEDICATIONS
1. Ecotrin 1 p.o. b.i.d. with meals.
2. Keflex 500 mg p.o. q.i.d. x 4 days.
3. Iron sulfate 325 mg p.o. b.i.d.

PLAN
The patient is to see me again in two weeks. She will call if symptoms recur.

Appendix B

The Mark of Zorro

Robert L. Love

The following does not constitute legal, accounting, or other professional service. If legal advice or other expert assistance is advisable or required, the services of a professional should be sought.

In colonial Spanish California, there was but one Zorro:

> That gay renegade carved
>   a "Z" with his blade,
> A "Z" that stands for Zorro.

No one had to worry about the authenticity of his signature, or whether an imposter had been masquerading as Zorro.

If alive today, Zorro would be appalled at the amount of forgery, backdating, tampering with transcripts—need I go on?—occurring in medical reports. He might even be tempted to drag the tip of his blade across the bottoms of some of the most egregious offenders.

Alas, that option is not one available to modern medical transcriptionists. Instead of blades, you have documentation and audit trails ... not nearly as gallant and romantic, but nonetheless effective.

Why do you need an effective documentation procedure? Why worry about audit trails?

- Have any of your transcribed reports ever been altered after leaving your possession?

- Has an incorrect date of dictation or review and approval ever been included in the dictation you receive or the report you generate?

- Have you ever been given dictation by one individual, who dictates the name of another at the end of the tape?

- Has the narrative ever been changed after the fact for purposes other than medical accuracy?

- Have you ever been asked to alter (falsify) any part of a report?

If none of the above has ever happened to you (and you have no concern about it happening in the future), you can stop reading this article. For the rest of us, however, documentation and audit trails are a professional necessity.

What do you need to document? What you received, what the content was, what you did with it, and what it said when it left your possession.

What is an audit trail? The "who's and where's" of documentation: who delivered it to you, who worked on it, who quality-checked it, who in your organization delivered it, and who took custody of it.

Keeping the recording from which you transcribe or the transcript itself is not possible. Instead, keep an audit trail.

The importance of audit trails

In court, it is called the "chain of custody." In some instances, you will not be able to offer evidence unless you can establish the evidence's pedigree—the chain of custody.

Why is an audit trail important? Because, speaking empirically, there is no way to prove the absolute (veracity and integrity) without being able to document the entire life of the report/evidence and the fact that at no time whatsoever was there even the remotest possibility that the report/evidence could have fallen into someone else's hands. Note that we are talking about remotest *possibility,* not remotest *probability.*

Evidence is completely excluded thousands of times a day from America's courts because an adequate chain of custody could not be established by the people offering the evidence.

So, how long should you keep such documentation? After checking on your state's limitations statutes, determine what you believe is a reasonable period of time. Then double that and add fifty years to it. With that, you are probably covered.

The point is to be prepared with complete and accurate information in the event it becomes necessary to defend yourself in a court of law.

The errant participant

… or physician … or supervisor. It can be anyone. They just have to request that you do something which at the very least is unprofessional. These people give little thought to the shared covenant with the patient, medical practice acts, accreditation standards, and requirements.

How do you handle them? If they are acting out of ignorance, you enlighten them. But if they are acting out of expediency and—worse yet—fully cognizant of what they are asking, do you refuse to do as they request? What if it is your supervisor and such an act could cost you your job, or a client and you could lose the account?

- If possible, try explaining why it should not be done, explaining the benefits of sticking to the straight and narrow.

- If that doesn't work, ask that they put their request in writing.

- If neither of the first two suggestions prove successful, or if you are not in a position to explain or challenge them, document the sequence of events, the people involved, the content of the conversation, and secure this material.

The bottom line is that you must take the most proactive steps possible to protect yourself, both short- and long-term.

Reprinted from "Legal Briefs," JAAMT, Vol. 12, No. 4, July-August 1993, p. 22. Copyright 1993, AAMT, Modesto, CA.

Appendix C

When Did "CMT" Become "MD"?

Robert L. Love

The following does not constitute legal, accounting, or other professional service. If legal advice or other expert assistance is advisable or required, the services of a professional should be sought.

It didn't, it hasn't, and it won't. But, every time you "drop in" a physician's "signature on file" or "electronic signature" to a medical report that a physician has not and will not read, you are practicing medicine without a license. You, the medical transcriptionist, are playing doctor and certifying not only that the report has been transcribed as accurately as possible given the raw material provided but also that (1) the treatment evidenced by the report accurately reflects not only what was dictated but also what actually occurred, and (2) that treatment was, under the circumstances involved, appropriate and proper.

The biggest problem with physician electronic signatures, etc., is not the huge amount of liability you assume. The biggest problem is that it violates the patient's trust and expectation that each professional in the healthcare chain will do the absolute best that he or she can do to render the best care available.

Such practices, as indicated above, violate most medical practice acts. They also violate applicable JCAHO standards and accreditation requirements.

I do not believe that most physicians, hospital executives, or health information managers are consciously attempting to provoke such massive problems when they attempt to force a transcriptionist to medically certify a report. I believe that most of them are one or more of the following: busy, self-important, lazy, uninformed, careless, stupid. Take your pick, but please don't choose to act in the same manner.

It is a very poorly kept secret that many physicians hate to review and certify/sign reports. Some have to be threatened with expulsion from medical staffs in order to insure compliance. Hospital and clinic administrative staffs hate to confront physicians over these circumstances. They also hate to have payment denied for incomplete reports or suffer the indignity of JCAHO accreditation site visits at times of incomplete reports.

Some of these people attempt to "shame" transcriptionists into these practices. "What about all that 'quality' you tell me about ... your checking, flagging, etc.? Don't you really do that?"

Sure you do. But, let's remember what you contract to provide: a report that has been transcribed as accurately and timely as possible given the raw material provided. You have not contracted to provide legal certification that the raw material is factually accurate and medically appropriate.

I understand that AAMT is developing a position statement on this issue. I applaud and support this effort, and ask you to do the same.

Reprinted from "Legal Briefs," JAAMT, Vol. 12, No. 3, May-June 1993, p. 26. Copyright 1993, AAMT, Modesto, CA.

Appendix D

What's Wrong With This Picture?

Claudia Tessier, CAE, CMT, RRA

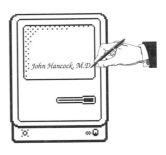

My executive message this issue is lengthier and "heavier" than most have been: so much so that we have made it a feature article. Its topic was introduced in our new legal column in the May-June 1993 *JAAMT*: the proliferating practice of autoauthentication of patient records by the dictator at the time of dictation, or its alternative, the "dropping in" of electronic signatures by the medical transcriptionist. These practices are or will or should be of concern to each of you.

The American Health Information Management Association (AHIMA) is a leading proponent of these practices. In its April issue, the AHIMA journal provides definitions related to these practices:

Electronic signature is a generic definition for any method of establishing authorship to a statement or document by the use of electricity. Electronic signatures may be initiated by computer key, voice, fingerprint, or fax.

Autosignature ... uses a dictation system's unique physician identification as the computer key signature for authenticating dictated patient health record documents.

Among the reasons AHIMA and others cite for promoting autosignature and nonclinician use of clinicians' electronic signatures on dictated reports are (1) reducing the physicians' burden (MDs won't have to sign reports themselves anymore); (2) reducing the health information managers' burden (HIMs won't have to run after physicians to sign records anymore, and they won't have so many incomplete records because reports have not been authenticated); (3) the computer-based patient record (CPR) cannot be readily implemented if we don't relax the authentication requirements; and (4) costs can be cut by eliminating the requirement for physicians (and other caregivers) to authenticate their own records in a timely manner.

What's wrong with this picture? Almost everything! It places the convenience of MDs and HIMs, as well as technology and cost-cutting measures, before patients' rights to quality care—and passes the buck of the legal burden to the MT (or anyone else they can give it to). Yes, I include quality documentation of patient care as an essential component of patients' rights. Any HIM text will tell you that the purposes of patient care documentation include facilitating continuity and improvement of patient care. If future care is to be at least partially determined by past care, as documented in the record (computer-based or not), then that documentation is going to influence subsequent care. If the documentation is inaccurate, it could have drastic implications for all parties concerned, most importantly the patient.

The demand and expectation for quality in patient care documentation must increase, not decrease, in the world of computer-based patient records. With a single, longitudinal record, the impact of inaccuracy will increase exponentially as past errors lead to present errors that in turn lead to future errors, some potentially lethal. The 1993 MT week slogan, "Medical Transcription: Where Quality Counts," says it all. But it takes more than MTs to assure accuracy; we can say our transcripts are accurate, but we cannot say the dictation was—or that the care documented was the care given—and therein lies the problem.

It is false logic to state that timely implementation of the computer-based patient record requires relaxation of authentication requirements. What we need from technology is what we must seek and demand; when we start settling for what we can get instead of what we need, we're encouraging the tail to wag the dog even more than it already does.

Then there is the argument that costs must be cut and relaxing authentication requirements will do this. What happened to the healthcare system's move toward total quality management (TQM)? Here we have one of the oldest and most inadequate excuses for doing something wrong: it costs less. This is in direct opposition to a basic TQM tenet and almost anyone's experience: If you want to do things at less cost, do them right the first time so that you don't have to pay to have them re-done or pay for the consequences of errors.

Somehow, we must persuade the decision-makers that medical documentation requires a process of checks and balances and that medical transcriptionists are an important part of that process. One attorney I talked to, who is particularly frustrated by the eagerness with which caregivers and HIMs are embracing autoauthentication and noncaregiver use of caregivers' electronic signatures, predicts that it will take major courtroom cases to get their attention. Attorneys will be eager to read the reports that caregivers haven't read or authenticated appropriately.

One suggestion for speeding along the computer-based patient record is to have MDs and other caregivers do their own entries, thereby eliminating the need for MTs. There are some major problems with this logic: If MDs don't want to take the time to review and sign their own reports, how can they be persuaded to do their own entries? (Some have suggested paying them to do their own keyboarding, which can't help but make an MT wonder: Will they be paid by the line, the character, the report, or the hour? Maybe instead, there should be talk of paying them to sign their own reports.)

Then, of course, there is voice recognition technology, which would provide what too many think they get (and want) now: verbatim transcription. If voice recognition technology is to be successful, it must be married to the editorial skills of medical editors, a.k.a. medical transcriptionists. Indeed, I've never understood why researchers and developers in voice recognition have not seen the logic of involving MTs; they and we and improved patient care documentation would move forward a lot faster. Another proposed solution is voice storage: store the dictation instead of transcribing it; then future users can listen to it rather than read its translation. This scenario might be the most effective for stimulating recognition for MTs: While it takes less time to dictate than to transcribe, it takes more time to listen than to read, and retention is reduced, meaning errors in recall are likely to be high, and listening will have to be repeated. And then there is the nightmare of retrieval. I don't think it would take long for users to begin to demand transcripts, and guess whom they would turn to?

Encouraging autoauthentication and electronic signatures by other than the author presents convincing evidence that the ignorance about medical transcription is not only widespread but excessive—and potentially dangerous to patients. MTs have been frustrated for years by the view from nontranscriptionists that transcription is a clerical task, "You just transcribe what the doctor says, don't you? Anyone who can type can do that." The frustration is the result of many factors, not the least of which is the insult of dismissing the MTs' special knowledge and its critical value to quality patient care documentation. This in turn leads to inadequate pay, inappropriate job classifications and titles, and low self-esteem, so that too many MTs continue to accept their lot rather than try to change it.

Many MTs have shared their frustrations with us. Most (but in truth, not all) are in work settings in which their supervisors, managers, or service owners are not MTs. We at AAMT have also experienced these frustrations, some personally when we were practicing MTs (certainly I could tell some horror stories of my own), and we all have experienced them indirectly as we represent the MT profession in the wider community. When we hear your individual horror stories, our frustration is heightened because we cannot intervene directly on your behalf. AAMT and its leaders cannot represent you personally in your individual workplace, but we can and do represent your profession and speak to these issues in the wider healthcare community.

As I have discussed previously, one of the ways in which we do this is through the establishment of strategic alliances. These constitute a form of networking with other associations, agencies, and organizations. As with any networking activity, not every contact creates a positive relationship. Some never work, some keep going through courtesy exchanges of information, some develop strong mutual benefits, and sometimes, just when we least expect it, things click.

We want you to know about some important relationships that are developing for AAMT, for the profession of medical transcription, and thus, for you. When AAMT became aware of the push being made to encourage adoption of policies for autoauthentication and for electronic signatures being done by MTs and others not directly delivering patient care, we recognized immediately that these practices would put not only transcriptionists, but also physicians, other caregivers, institutions, and, most important, patients, at risk. And we began to explore the issue with other associations and agencies. As a result, we've gotten our foot in some doors—while other doors, quite frankly, have been shut in our face. But we will keep trying.

Let me tell you about our progress to date. As previously noted, we brought the matter to your attention in the last *JAAMT* through our new legal column. At the recent MTIA (Medical Transcription Industry Alliance) conference, at which adoption of these practices was discussed by a panel including HIMs and MTSOs (medical transcription service owners), we spoke out against it, providing background information and rationale that caused an attorney to express second thoughts about it.

When we failed in our efforts to be included in a meeting between AHIMA and JCAHO (Joint Commission on Accreditation of Healthcare Organizations) at which they were to discuss the JCAHO position requiring that physicians and other caregivers authenticate their own records after reviewing them, we wrote to JCAHO urging them to sustain their position. Our letters to JCAHO and other parties include the following key points:

> … Medical transcriptionists are medical language specialists who transcribe dictated patient reports so that they are as complete, clear, consistent, and correct as possible, given the information provided by the dictating physician or other caregiver. Medical transcription responsibilities include correcting English usage, discriminating among soundalike terms, researching new terminology, correcting spelling, and expanding abbreviations to make them clear to the reader.

> While medical transcriptionists can attest to the accuracy of their transcription, it is a different matter to authenticate that the information provided by the dictating physician or other caregiver is accurate. Because medical transcriptionists are not clinicians and because dictators are not always accurate, it is inappropriate for the MT to authenticate reports. Sometimes dictators do not identify themselves. Since MTs may transcribe for a multitude of dictators, they may not recognize each dictator's voice. The MT cannot even be certain that the dictated report relates to the patient identified by the physician.

> We acknowledge that it is difficult to assure that physicians authenticate each report. But assigning authentication responsibility to MTs is inappropriate, and we are concerned that doing so places the medical transcriptionist, the dictator, and the healthcare institution in a position of potential legal risk.

> More important, such practices place the patient at risk. Authentication communicates a degree of confidence in the content of the patient's record that only the direct caregiver can provide. Only on review of the transcribed

report can the caregiver confidently assure that the content is accurate and complete and that it pertains to the appropriate patient. ...

Since writing, we have been assured that the JCAHO position remains intact. They have disapproved the use of autosignature as complying with their standards because autosignature does not prove the author reviewed the report and confirmed the accuracy of its content. Furthermore, they have interpreted the computer key signature as requiring real-time, on-screen review of the transcribed report by the physician who has coded access to the computer system.

JCAHO representatives have referred to us inquiries about the issue, and they have advised those making the inquiries that the AAMT position is consistent with theirs. Further, they recommend reading the legal column in our May-June journal. Additionally, JCAHO has invited us to become a part of their liaison network.

For your information, JCAHO standards that speak to autoauthentication include the following (emphases ours).

MR3
Medical records are confidential, secure, current, **authenticated,** legible, and complete.

MR3.4
The quality of the medical record depends in part on the timeliness, meaning-fulness, **authentication,** and legibility of the informational content.

MR3.4.1. Entries in medical records are made only by individuals given this right as specified in hospital and medical staff policies.

MR3.4.2. All entries in the record are dated and **authenticated, and a method is established to identify the authors of entries.**

MR3.4.2.1. Identification may include written signatures, initials, or **computer key.**

MR3.4.2.2. When rubberstamp signatures are authorized, **the individual whose signature the stamp represents** places in the administrative offices of the hospital a signed statement to the effect that he/she **is the only one who has the stamp and is the only one who will use it.**

MR3.4.2.2.1. There is **no delegation of the use** of such a stamp to another individual.

MR3.4.3. **The parts of the medical record that are the responsibility of the medical practitioner are authenticated by the practitioner.**

In our letter to JCAHO, we emphasized that an electronic signature should be treated much as a rubber-stamp signature: only the individual whose signature it represents should use it. Indeed they require that the physician be the only one who uses the computer code to access computer entries and that s/he personally enter the computer key to affix her/his signature.

We have also communicated our concerns about autoauthentication and electronic signatures to the U.S. Department of Health and Human Services (HHS), whose prompt response assured us that they agreed that "medical transcriptionists should not be required to authenticate medical records for the reasons given in your letter." HHS noted that autoauthentication and misuse of electronic signatures are inconsistent with the Medicare requirement and that they "are currently assessing the extent of this problem and will take appropriate action." Their relevant policies, include 42 CFR 482.24(c) (again, emphases ours):

(c) Standard: Content of record. The medical record must contain information to justify admission and continued hospitalization, support the diagnosis, and describe the patient's progress and response to medications.

(1) All entries must be legible and complete, and **must be authenticated and dated promptly by the person (identified by name and discipline) who is responsible for ordering, providing, or evaluating the service furnished.**

(i) **The author of each entry must be identified and must authenticate his or her entry.**

(ii) **Authentication may include signatures, written initials or computer entry.**

We have also communicated our concerns, with rationale, to other groups, such as the American Hospital Association and the American Bar Association, and we will be expressing these concerns to the AMA and to the Computer-based Patient Record Institute (CPRI), where AHIMA is placing the topic on the agenda. At a recent American Medical Informatics Association (AMIA) meeting, we spoke up and out at every opportunity. Because we are particularly concerned that AHIMA is in favor of autoauthentication and electronic signature usage by other than the caregiver, we have expressed our concerns directly to them as well, urging their caution and offering our assistance in addressing authentication problems.

Other communications are planned, through correspondence, articles, meetings, etc. And a position paper on autoauthentication and electronic signatures will be presented to AAMT's 1993 House of Delegates for their adoption.

Individual hospitals have been in contact with us through their attorneys, HIMs, or MT supervisors, and as a result many have made or are considering changes in practices related to autoauthentication and electronic signatures. Unfortunately, some MTs who have contacted us about these practices being imposed on them are afraid of losing their jobs if they protest or bring AAMT's position to the attention of their supervisors, managers, or MT service owners. This again brings TQM to mind: Among its basic tenets are those that call for eliminating fear in the workplace and involving those most knowledgeable about a process in decisions relating to that process. (As an aside, I can't resist telling you that some MTs have shared their institution's [pseudo] policies with us, policies that on paper appear to be in conformity with JCAHO practices but in practice bypass the caregiver when it comes to authentication and direct the MT to drop in the signature at the time of transcription.)

MTs and AAMT have been cut out of the loop in too many instances, and we are doing all we can to get back in. Clearly, of great concern to us over this matter is the potential legal risk to the medical transcriptionist. But we must put the patient first. It will be so easy for proponents of autoauthentication and electronic signatures to point their fingers at AAMT and MTs and challenge us. In fact, some already have: "You mean you're not as good as you've been saying you are all these years. You mean you're not ready to stand behind the quality of your work." Beware of these arguments. They beg the question—and they demonstrate others' rampant ignorance about medical transcription.

Our response, and yours, must be: We stand behind the quality of our transcription. But we can't confirm that the patient named by the dictator is appropriately matched with the report dictated—or any part of it. We can't be certain that the dictator has appropriately identified himself or herself. We don't profess to be clinicians. We do profess to be language specialists. We do our best, with what is given us, to make our transcripts as complete, correct, clear, consistent, and readable as possible.

Only the authenticator can attest to a record's validity, and we agree with the JCAHO **definition of authenticator: "to prove authorship,** for example, by written signature, identifiable initials, or computer key." Medical transcriptionists are not authors, we are editors. Interestingly, Canadian transcriptionists speak of authors instead of dictators. Perhaps we would be wise to change our terminology so as to draw attention to the reality of the situation. Physicians and other caregivers are not just dictating reports, they are authoring legal statements.

References

Correspondence to AAMT dated April 1993 from Health Care Financing Administration, Department of Health & Human Services.

Feste, L., "Electronic Signature—As It Is Today," *Journal of AHIMA.* (Chicago: AHIMA 1993), Vol. 64, No. 4, pp. 18–19.

Joint Commission on Accreditation of Healthcare Organizations, Accreditation Manual for Hospitals (Oakbrook Terrace: JCAHO, 1993), pp. 50–51, 219.

Love, R.L., "When Did 'CMT' Become 'MD?'" *JAAMT,* May-June 1993, p. 26.
"Update on AHIMA Action Regarding Electronic Authentication," April 1993
  (Chicago: AHIMA 1993).

Meetings, including:

  AAMT Supervisors and Managers Conference, April 1993, Denver, CO.
  MTIA Conference, April 1993, San Francisco, CA.
  AMIA Conference, May 1993, St. Louis, MO.

AAMT Position Paper: Providers' Signatures

Issue

Delegation of authority to affix healthcare providers' signatures (by electronic, rubber-stamp, or other means) to patient records.

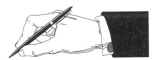

This position statement addresses concerns related to the practice by physicians and other healthcare providers of delegating to the medical transcriptionist the authority to affix providers' signature to patient records.

Issue summary

Some healthcare institutions have established policies that allow physicians and other healthcare providers to delegate to the medical transcriptionist the authority to affix providers' signatures (by electronic, rubber-stamp, or other means) to patient records.

Reasons cited for establishing these policies and encouraging these practices include (1) reducing the healthcare providers' burden of signing reports; (2) reducing the burden of health information managers and others for assuring that providers sign reports; (3) reducing the numbers of incomplete records; (4) accelerating the implementation of computer-based patient records; and (5) reducing costs associated with requirements that providers review and sign their own records in a timely manner.

Current standards of the Joint Commission on Accreditation of Healthcare Organizations (JCAHO) and Medicare guidelines of the Healthcare Financing Administration (HCFA) of the U.S. Department of Health and Human Services (HHS) require that signatures, electronic or other, be done by the practitioner and not be delegated. AAMT is concerned by efforts to persuade JCAHO and HCFA to change their requirements.

Some institutions have policies that direct medical transcription employees, independent contractors, and services to affix the provider's signature as each transcript is completed. Others have documented policies that reflect compliance with JCAHO and HCFA, but implementation of these policies allows delegation of authority to affix signatures.

AAMT position

The American Association for Medical Transcription supports the JCAHO standards and HCFA guidelines that permit the use of electronic signatures by physicians and other caregivers and require that signatures (electronic or other) be affixed by the author of each entry and not be delegated.

AAMT recommendations

AAMT recommends that communications be directed to associations, government agencies, physicians, hospital administrators, health information managers, medical transcription service owners, supervisors, managers, etc., clarifying the roles and responsibilities of the medical transcriptionist/medical language specialist as editor of medical documents and of the physician/dictator as author of medical documents.

Medical transcriptionists can attest to the quality of their transcription—that it is complete, correct, clear, and consistent as possible based on the dictation provided. But medical transcriptionists cannot attest to the accuracy of the dictation itself, including but not limited to the identity of the dictating provider and of the patient, the dates given, the history and treatment recorded, and the conclusions reached. Only the direct caregiver can attest to the accuracy of patient care documentation.

AAMT recommends that the patient be of primary concern to all parties when any signature policies are established. The patient's record will be a primary source for future care as well as documentation for legal, reimbursement, and statistical purposes. Thus, AAMT recommends that policies assure that the content accuracy of the patient record is the responsibility of the healthcare provider and that they specifically state that delegation of the authority to affix one's signature is not appropriate or allowed.

Position summary

Medical transcriptionists are medical language specialists who transcribe dictated patient reports. They interpret and edit raw data (dictation) in as complete, clear, consistent, and correct a manner as possible.

Medical transcriptionists can attest to the accuracy of their transcription; they cannot attest to the accuracy of the dictation on which it is based.

Patient care and well-being are at risk if proper attention is not given by the healthcare provider to the content of the patient record before the provider's signature is affixed. The provider's signature communicates accuracy of record content that only the provider can give; thus, delegation of authority to affix signatures is inappropriate and should not be allowed.

Adopted by AAMT House of Delegates, August 4, 1993.
Copyright 1993, AAMT, Modesto, CA.

Appendix F

AAMT Explores Quality and Quantity Issues

In a series of meetings initiated by AAMT with the American Health Information Management Association (AHIMA) and the Medical Transcription Industry Alliance (MTIA), key industry representatives are discussing issues and concerns regarding the business of medical transcription. Participants have agreed not to set or enforce standards, and each organization remains free to act independently. Discussions to date have focused on quality and quantity.

QUALITY

Ideal characteristics of quality patient care documentation as they relate to the dictation/transcription process include:

Complete—All required, desired, and relevant information is documented.

Consistent—All information is consistent within each report and with the remainder of the patient record.

Clear—The information can be readily understood for patient care, reimbursement, statistical, research, and legal purposes.

Correct—The documentation is accurate in content and presentation.

Concurrent—The documentation is dictated, transcribed, authenticated, and incorporated into the patient record in a timely manner.

Credible—The documentation system provides realistic means for achieving quality, including appropriate opportunities and methods for corrections.

Confidential—The patient's rights to confidentiality and privacy are protected throughout the documentation process (dictation and transcription, storage, maintenance, and usage).

Concise—The report is well organized and succinct.

Commitment—The report reflects a commitment to professionalism and quality.

Collaboration—The report demonstrates appropriate use of references and other resources necessary to prepare a high-quality document.

Communication—The report effectively documents patient care.

CQI (continuous quality improvement)—The report demonstrates continuing efforts to improve the process and content of patient care documentation.

QUANTITY

Quantitative units that can be clearly and consistently applied and verified within medical transcription include:

Character—Any letter, number, symbol, or function key necessary for the final appearance and content of a document, including the space bar, carriage return, underscore, bold, and any character contained within a macro, header, or footer. *AAMT prefers the character as the basic unit of measure, where such measures are appropriate.*

Word—Five (5) characters. *Total character count can be converted to words by dividing total character count by the specified number of characters in a word, in this instance 5.*

Line—Sixty-five (65) characters. *The total number of lines for reporting purposes is determined by dividing total characters by the specified number of characters in a line, in this instance 65. Margins may vary, resulting in gross lines of varying numbers of characters. (See "Gross line of transcription" below.)*

Our comments below demonstrate the inadequacies of other units used to measure transcription.

Keystroke—The strike of a single key. *Measures "input" only, reducing a macro to entry strokes rather than meaningful output terms.*

Gross line of transcription—A line of print with one or more printed characters. *Obsolete and inconsistent; a gross line may consist of a single character or as many characters as will fit between the margins. (See "Line" above.)*

Minute of dictation—A measure of access time to a dictation unit or system. *The definition of access time may vary among units/systems, so that a minute of dictation is not consistent among units/systems.*

Page of transcription—One side of any size sheet of paper with one or more printed characters on it. *Inconsistent since the paper can be of any size, with any number of printed characters.*

Still other units of measure are rarely used (*e.g.,* report); are difficult to define clearly, consistently, and verifiably (*e.g.,* byte); or already have established meanings (*e.g.,* ASCII text byte).

QUALITY COUNTS IN MEDICAL TRANSCRIPTION

Medical transcription is not simply the striking of a series of keys to create a string of characters, words, lines, pages, or reports. Rather, it is the process by which raw data in the form of dictation are translated into meaningful communication for the purpose of documenting patient care. This translation and the fund of knowledge behind it demonstrate that quality counts in medical transcription far more than quantity.

Reprinted from an AAMT news release dated March 1994. Copyright 1994, AAMT, Modesto, CA.

Appendix G

Can You Keep a Secret?

Pat Forbis, CMT

Confidentiality as it pertains to a patient's right to privacy does not exist; there are only individuals who hold confidences about patient information.

Confidentiality of the medical record and protection of the patient's right to privacy is an issue that is of concern to every recordkeeper. Webster's definition of confidential is simply that it is "marked by intimacy or willingness to confide," and it refers the reader to the words secret and private, both of which state "something kept from the knowledge of others or shared only confidentially with a few." Privileged (as in privileged information), on the other hand, is defined in stronger terms, "not subject to the usual rules ... not subject to disclosure in a court of law."

There are laws that were written specifically to protect patients' privacy. Federal laws speak to the protection of the patient's privacy, but there are exceptions to them. State statutes reflect confidentiality laws, but there are exceptions to them as well.

The American Medical Association (AMA) has a formal confidentiality statement. Included in the two-paragraph statement is the following: "The physician should not reveal confidential communications or information without the express consent of the patient, unless required to do so by law." There are those exceptions again.

The hippocratic oath admonishes physicians in part, "All that may come to my knowledge in the exercise of my profession or outside of my profession or in daily commerce with men, which ought not to be spread abroad, I will keep secret and will never reveal." Hippocrates did not make exceptions. I suspect his concern was one of ethics and not of legality. The father of medicine probably had few record-keeping concerns.

In 1984 the American Medical Record Association (AMRA) issued an 11-page document that established specific guidelines regarding confidentiality of the patient record. Three years later an additional 13-page document was released that speaks to confidentiality as it pertains to AIDS-related patient records.

Healthcare facilities, whether major medical centers or private offices, have internal policies regarding patient confidentiality. Most facilities require that personnel sign agreements ensuring commitment to those policies. Generally, the agreements quote portions of one law or another and cite the penalty that could accompany indiscretion. Clearly no exceptions.

What about the exceptions? To what extent is it acceptable to release information about patients; the information patients are encouraged to give because they are assured it is safe to do so? Nowhere is it stated how many people can have access to confidential information before it is no longer confidential.

The court can subpoena patient records. The court can direct disclosure of confidential records when reporting child abuse, socially transmitted disease, AIDS, and communicable disease, drug abuse, criminal acts, harm to oneself or others. If a jury is seated, the record is usually enlarged so it can be easily read from a distance. You may also be required by either federal or state law to release confidential information during inspections and for credentialing purposes. There is also disclosure upon request and disclosure for medical research.

The law states that in order for "others" to obtain information about the patient, the patient must consent or authorize release of information in his/her record. In order to obtain treatment in most healthcare facilities patients are required to sign a disclosure statement. The disclosure statement allows additional release of information to insurance carriers to investigate as they deem necessary the patient's medical record. Oh, yes, it's also permissible to provide patient information to the statistical center that provides information to insurance companies when they investigate individuals for possible pre-existing conditions to determine whether or not a policy applicant warrants consideration for insurance coverage.

It appears that there was a time not so long ago when the expectation of confidentiality was more realistic than it is today. In the years BT (before technology) a breach of confidentiality could be tracked more times than not. Enter technology with accessibility to everything and everybody within minutes. Controlled management of sophisticated technology systems is difficult and lack of confidentiality is absolute. Ethical software has yet to be introduced.

Technology has focused on designing programs that allow computer access by code only. The concept is that the individual who possesses the code is the only person privy to the patient's information. Ongoing concerns, revisions in design, and workshops that answer questions from anxious users confirm skeptics' belief that technology jeopardizes patient confidentiality. In a recent article on optical storage and its implementation, a senior manager of a Chicago consulting company notes, "Multiple access to medical records from multiple locations for multiple purposes, will eliminate record contention."

Technological capability is awesome. Telephones and modems allow transmission of anything to anyone. One technology expert states, "I believe an electronic medical record can be developed to meet the ever increasing demands of medical records. This system would have total connectivity to serve multiple departments along with key functions of abstracting, editing, coding, chart tracking, chart deficiency, and management reporting." Impressive.

In terms of medical transcription dictation, patient information is volleyed from any point in the U.S. and back again. When a transcriptionist finishes a document and sends it into the computer network or modem, control of that record's confidentiality is gone. Many transcriptionists don't even see the printed document these days or know who takes their work from the printer.

Confidentiality and the patient's so-called right to privacy are a curious study. When is the information no longer confidential? When the physician dictates about the patient, a third party shares the confidence. When the third person transcribes it, it is distributed to "appropriate parties." How many parties? Who knows. Perhaps a more appropriate and more ethical approach to patient confidentiality would be to employ a restricted list. The list would simply inform recordkeepers who isn't an appropriate party, for example: Do not reveal the contents of the patient's medical record to the patient's next door neighbor. The next door neighbor is one of the few "others" left who is not an exception to the patient's right to privacy.

And, wouldn't it be more in the patient's best interest to provide him/her a list that reveals who receives privileged information? Would that approach be uncomfortable for those who seek release of information and those who release it? If such a list were necessary, I suspect "appropriate party" would be more carefully scrutinized.

Reprinted from "Impressions," JAAMT, Vol. 10, No. 2, March-April 1991, pp. 8–9. Copyright 1991, AAMT, Modesto, CA.

Healthcare Reform and Confidentiality

Kathleen Frawley, JD, RRA

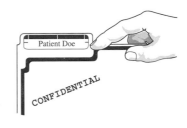

O ne of the most important aspects of the relationship between a patient and a healthcare provider is the provider's duty to maintain the confidentiality of health information. The historical origin of a physician's obligation is found in the Oath of Hippocrates, written between the sixth century B.C. and the first century A.D. The Oath states "what I may see or hear in the course of treatment in regard to the life of men, which on no account one must spread abroad, I will keep to myself ..."

The American Medical Association, the American Hospital Association, and the American Health Information Management Association have all promulgated guidelines to address the confidentiality of health information.

The legal obligation of healthcare providers to maintain the confidentiality of health information derives from licensure laws and regulations, specific statutes and regulations on medical record confidentiality, Medicare's Conditions of Participation, standards of the Joint Commission on Accreditation of Healthcare Organizations (JCAHO), and court decisions.

Unfortunately, there is little uniformity among state licensure laws and regulations on the requirements for medical records, and much confusion remains over whether patient records may be created and stored in a computer-based format.

The recently released Office of Technology Assessment (OTA) report, *Protecting Privacy in Computerized Medical Information,* found that current laws do not, in general, provide consistent, comprehensive protection of health information confidentiality. Focusing on the impact of computer technology, the report concluded that computerization reduces some concerns about privacy of health information while increasing others. The report highlights the need for enactment of a comprehensive federal privacy law.

The public's concern about the confidentiality of health information was identified in a poll conducted by Louis Harris and Associates for Equifax, Inc. The results of the *Health Information Privacy Survey 1993* were released at a conference sponsored by the American Health Information Management Association (AHIMA) and Equifax in conjunction with the U.S. Office of Consumer Affairs on October 26, 1993. Senator Patrick Leahy (D-VT) and Representative Pete Stark (D-CA) and several panelists identified the need to address privacy of health information in any healthcare reform plan.

The survey found that a large majority of Americans (89%) believe reforming health care is one of the top domestic issues facing the nation today. Fifty-six percent (56%) indicated strong support for comprehensive federal legislation to protect the privacy of medical records as part of healthcare reform.

There was high agreement on what should be included in national privacy legislation. Ninety-six percent (96%) believe federal legislation should designate all personal medical information as sensitive and impose severe penalties for unauthorized disclosure. Ninety-five percent (95%) favor legislation that addresses individuals' rights to access their medical records and creating procedures for updating or correcting those records.

Currently, there is little uniformity among state licensure laws and regulations regarding confidentiality of health information. It has been recognized that there is a need for more uniformity among the 50 states. In recent years, the National Conference of Commissioners on Uniform State Laws developed the Uniform Health Care Information Act in an attempt to stimulate uniformity among states on healthcare information management issues. Presently, only two states, Montana and Washington, have enacted this model legislation. Clearly, efforts must be directed toward developing national standards on privacy and confidentiality.

Healthcare reform and the national information infrastructure

The development of the national information infrastructure is a key component of healthcare reform. Efforts to reform this country's healthcare delivery system will rely heavily on administrative simplification and computerization of health information to control costs, improve quality of care, and increase efficiency. The increasing need for data highlights the need for federal pre-emptive legislation to protect the confidentiality of health information.

In the Administration's Health Security Act (Title V, Subtitle B, Part 2), privacy of personal health information is addressed. The National Health Board would be established to develop and implement a health information system. Within two years of enactment of this Act, the National Health Board would be responsible for the development of privacy and security standards to address unauthorized disclosure and provide individuals with the right to access their personal health information. The Act requires that, within three years of enactment, the Board shall submit to the President and Congress a comprehensive legislative proposal, based on a Code of Fair Information Practices, to protect the privacy of individually identifiable health information.

There are a number of other bills which have been introduced in Congress to address the need for federal legislation. The Health Care Information Modernization and Security Act of 1993 (H.R. 3137) contains specific provisions to address privacy and to ensure the confidentiality of information. The Fair Health Information

Practices Act of 1994 establishes uniform, comprehensive federal rules governing the use and disclosure of identifiable health information about individuals.

It is critical that federal legislation be enacted to address the privacy of personal health information. Healthcare information is personal and sensitive information, that if improperly used or released, may cause harm to a patient and affect their ability to obtain employment or insurance. The movement of patients and their healthcare information across state lines, the development of electronic networks, and the emergence of multi-state providers and payors creates a compelling need for federal law governing the use and disclosure of healthcare information.

Reprinted from JAAMT, *Vol. 13, No. 3, May-June 1994, pp. 36, 38. Copyright 1994, AAMT, Modesto, CA.*

Electronic Monitoring: Outquotes and Thoughts

Claudia Tessier, CAE, CMT, RRA

What is electronic monitoring and what are its effects? Are legislative restrictions necessary to protect employees and the public? In an effort to explore the answers to these questions, we provide excerpts from a variety of sources, followed by a brief discussion of electronic monitoring in relation to medical transcription.

From 9to5, National Association of Working Women:

> Supervisors are now present in the very tools office workers use. Computers total the number of keystrokes per minute, errors and corrections per hour, and even the length of restroom breaks. The National Institute for Occupational Safety and Health estimates that two-thirds of computer operations are monitored.

> With the computerized workforce now approaching 50 million, as many as 26 million workers may be under electronic scrutiny.

> According to a 1993 survey by *Macworld* magazine, more than 20% of employers responding engage in searches of employee computer files or electronic mail. While this survey estimates that 20 million Americans may be subjected to computer monitoring (this number does not include telephone surveillance) only 18% of companies surveyed had a written policy on electronic privacy for workers.

> Employers are no longer monitoring the work; they are monitoring the workers.

According to 9to5, under The Privacy for Consumers and Workers Act proposed by Senator Paul Simon (D-IL) and Representative Pat Williams (D-MT),

> Employers would be required to give employees and job applicants written explanation of when and how monitoring is used, what information is collected, how it is interpreted and how this data may affect production standards and performance evaluations. …

Monitoring of bathrooms, locker rooms or dressing rooms would not be permitted. Employers would be not allowed to intentionally collect information not relevant to the employee's work. ...

Employees would be guaranteed reasonable opportunity to review all personal information and interpretation of the information collected by electronic monitoring. Employers who violate any provisions of the bill would risk injunctive action by the Secretary of Labor, civil penalties of up to $10,000 and private suits.

Macworld *magazine's July 1993 article on electronic monitoring highlighted "A Model Employment-Privacy Policy," including the following points:*

Employees know what electronic surveillance tools are used, and how management uses the collected data.

Employees participate in decisions about how and when electronic monitoring or searches take place. Monitoring data will not be the sole factor in evaluating employee performance.

Employees can inspect, challenge, and correct electronic records kept on their activities or files captured through electronic means.

Electronic monitoring guidelines recommended by Tekneckron Infoswitch Corporation include,

First and most importantly, the monitors must be monitored. No monitoring should exist without technology capable for monitoring the supervisor (i.e., the monitor), which means that any scoring system used for an employee must also include a scoring system for the monitor. ... This will insure not only fair recording of the data but strong confidence by the employee that the people monitoring cannot abuse their employees.

And finally, a sampling of quotes from The Electronic Sweatshop: How Computers are Transforming the Office of the Future into the Factory of the Past, *by Barbara Garson (Penguin Books, 1988):*

... counting keystrokes can't tell you anything unless you know what all that communication is about.

What's countable may not be what counts. The bean counters can count the keystrokes but the intangibles get lost. ... They measure the easily measurable things, but they can't even differentiate between a typo and a mistake that makes the letter nonsense.

Electronic monitoring is cheap, efficient and total … the computer can monitor every worker every minute.

Monitoring, measuring and routinizing are usually justified as means of reducing labor costs. The fact that they reduce people is supposedly incidental.

And what about electronic monitoring in relation to medical transcription? It may well be that counting keystrokes (or words, or lines, or pages, or whatever) is an appropriate means by which to measure the quantity of transcription, but what about the quality of that transcription—or the quality of the dictation on which it is based—or the quality of the equipment on which it was done—or the quality of the references to which the transcriptionist has access—or the quality of the work environment in which s/he works—and so on? Certainly, counting transcription keystrokes (or whatever) is misused when unreasonable efforts are made to reduce that count (and therefore the MT's pay) by discounting, for example, the spaces between words, or by expecting the simplest dictation to be transcribed at the same rate as the most difficult.

And then there is electronic monitoring that is used to record keyboard vs non-keyboard time (read *productive vs nonproductive time*). Whether the MT is using non-keyboard time for a rest break, for a restroom break, to research terminology, to help another MT, or for whatever reason, such electronic monitoring reduces all such "absences" to non-keyboard time, reduces the MT to electronic shackles, and reduces the monitor to a bean counter that cannot differentiate one bean from another in terms of size, shape, type, taste, quality, or purpose.

Are there appropriate uses of electronic monitoring in medical transcription? Of course, including measuring productivity, provided other parameters such as quality and the factors influencing both quality and quantity are considered. It is likewise reasonable to use electronic monitoring data for management purposes such as scheduling, planning, and budgeting, but even then, other factors must be taken into account, for even the best-laid plans of MT supervisors and service owners …

Electronic monitoring is not a demon. It is a tool, and like any other tool it can be appropriately or inappropriately used. Its misuse and abuse are the targets of protective legislation and guidelines for both employees and the public.

Reprinted from "Executive Message," JAAMT, Vol. 12, No. 6, November-December 1993, pp. 4–5. Copyright 1993, AAMT, Modesto, CA.

Appendix J

Straight from the Source's Mouth

Claudia Tessier, CAE, CMT, RRA

In a previous editorial titled "May the Source Be with You" (*JAAMT,* Fall 1987), I discussed the difficulties and frustrations medical transcriptionists encounter in trying to determine whether a particular eponymic term takes the possessive form or not. Because there was no standard or guideline, there was no consistent practice. Even AAMT's position on the use of the possessive form for eponymic terms in medical transcription was inconclusive and inconsistent: Our *Style Guide for Medical Transcription* directed that for diseases, syndromes, tests, reflexes, operations, etc., consult *Dorland's, Stedman's,* or *Current Medical Information & Terminology,* or use the dictating physician's preference; for eponymic names of surgical instruments, do not use the possessive form.

I suggested that AAMT, as the recognized authority of medical transcription practices, state emphatically: In medical transcription, do not use the possessive form with eponyms. Of the few who reacted, most were pro, a few were con. The latter said that AAMT shouldn't set a language rule and MTs should continue to be guided by usage. This begs the question: At worst, it reduces MTs to the usage of each of the many physicians whose dictation they transcribe, thereby leading to inaccuracies and inconsistencies. At best, MTs are left to determine acceptable usage, and they come back again to the question of "whose usage?" An endless loop.

So our frustrations and difficulties persisted, particularly as we at AAMT continued to prepare education and reference materials for the profession. Finally, with the publication of AAMT's *Exploring Transcription Practices: Radiology Module* this year, we revised our guideline regarding eponyms. The following note from that module is repeated here for all readers:

> **Eponyms:** With this publication, AAMT is dropping the use of the possessive form with eponyms in medical transcription. Until now, there has been no consistent stylistic standard regarding this matter, and medical transcriptionsts have been guided on an eponym-by-eponym basis by the reference books consulted, dictators' usage, or each medical transcriptionist's preferences.
>
> Medical dictionaries, word books, and style manuals have been inadequate guides for the inclusion or exclusion of the possessive with eponyms. Even such highly regarded references as *Dorland's* or *Stedman's* medical dictionaries are inconsistent and incomplete. They vary both internally and with one another, and they do not include many of the eponymic terms confronted in medical transcription.

So, for consistency in medical transcription, AAMT recommends the deletion of the possessive form with eponyms and designates this as the preferred stylistic choice for transcribed medical records. For those who may be uncomfortable with this shift from tradition, AAMT acknowledges that to continue to be guided by *Dorland's* or other appropriate medical references is an acceptable alternative practice.

Some will welcome AAMT's guideline on eponyms, others will ignore it, others will reject it. No doubt some will question our authority in the matter, but that authority is clear: As the professional association for medical transcriptionists, AAMT is the appropriate body to speak for the profession, to speak about the profession, and to speak to the profession's practitioners.

Our guideline is both well reasoned and reasonable. It applies to medical transcription—our area of expertise and authority. We do not object or question that different guidelines may apply to different applications, e.g., manuscript preparation: let those with expertise and authority in those areas set guidelines for such usage. We sought the expertise of other sources in designing the guideline, but we found those sources wanting. That should come as no surprise. Those sources do not understand the questions, needs, and demands of the medical transcriptionist on the job. Finally, we designated the preferred form for medical transcription, but we allowed for alternate acceptable forms.

In its simplest form, AAMT's guidelines on eponyms is just as it was proposed in 1987: "In medical transcription, do not use the possessive form with eponyms." No longer need you check multiple sources. No longer need you question inconsistencies within a single reference or among several references. No longer need you question the variable usages among physicians. No longer need you develop your own list of the most commonly used eponyms and your conclusions based on your individual research.

Finally you have a consistent, reasonable standard for guidance. And when asked, "Who says?" just say your source is your association, your profession's association, the American Association for Medical Transcription.

Appendix K

Errors, Omissions, and the MT

Robert L. Love

The following does not constitute legal, accounting, or other professional service. If legal advice or other expert assistance is advisable or required, the services of a professional should be sought.

Errors and omissions" is an insurance industry term describing professional liability insurance. It got this name as shorthand for the conditions which can create professional malpractice liability. Become familiar with it.

What are some examples of "errors and omissions"?

- Doing something incorrectly, thereby causing damage to another who had a legal right to depend on your doing it correctly = *error.*

- Doing something that another had a legal right to depend on your **not** doing = *error.*

- Not doing something, thereby causing damage to another who had a legal right to depend on your doing what you failed to do = *omission.*

For liability to attach:

- You must have a legal duty to another person to do or to not do something.

- You must fail in your duty.

- The other person must suffer damage to person or property.

- The other person's damage must have been caused by your failure.

You may have a duty to someone for several reasons:

- You have an express agreement, written or oral.

- You have an implied agreement. These agreements are implied in law or fact. Example: You volunteer to provide your transcription services to a local hospice at no charge. A hospice patient dies prematurely because you transcribe *bella-donna* instead of *bottled water.* A defense of "I didn't charge; they didn't pay; I'm not responsible" will not be received well.

- Society imposes the duty. Examples: a state statute requiring certain licensure or certification, or maintenance of records for a certain period of time.

Once the existence of a duty is established, it must be defined. In contract disputes, did you or did you not perform as agreed? If you did not, is there sufficient legal justification for your nonperformance? Did the other party to the contract have to perform first and fail to do so, cancelling your obligation? Did you perform substantially as agreed?

Oftentimes, insurance company contracts specifically exclude any coverage for liability created voluntarily by their insureds. Examples:

- You have an "errors and omissions" policy. You deliberately mistype *belladonna*. The patient dies. The patient's estate sues the hospital, and the hospital sues you because of your error. Most insurance carriers will deny coverage because you deliberately created the exposure.

- You have an "errors and omissions" policy. You accidentally mistype *belladonna*. The patient dies. You are genuinely and sincerely overwrought by what the entire world knows is a pure accident on your behalf. The patient's estate sues the hospital, and the hospital makes a claim against you for indemnification pursuant to your written agreement to hold the hospital harmless and indemnify them from any and all claims. Your insurer denies the claim.

Wait a minute! The whole world knows that it was an accident! Why won't your professional liability policy pay? Because you voluntarily created the liability to the hospital when you signed a contract wherein you agreed to indemnify the hospital and hold it harmless.

There is a way to usually avoid this outcome. Do not agree to hold anyone harmless. Do not agree to indemnify anyone. Do agree to maintain certain minimum types and amounts of professional liability insurance and to provide proof of same to your client.

In disputes not involving a contract, were you obligated to render ordinary care? Extraordinary? Are you liable for negligence? Gross negligence? Or,

"That degree of skill and learning commonly applied under all the circumstances in the community by the average prudent reputable member of the medical transcription profession."

What is the "degree of skill and learning" in your hospital's community?

- Secretary able to type 100 WPM and willing to undergo on-the-job training?

- Two- or four-year college degree?

- Medical transcriptionist certification?

- Certain minimum continuing education requirements?

- A work environment with minimum criteria for space, equipment, library, work product auditing, and staffing ratios?

Is your local community's "degree of skill and learning" properly synchronized with the industry as a whole? Is there a disparity so great between the local and national environments that you could not, if called upon, defend local deficiencies?

Many reasons have been offered for medical transcriptionists not being concerned about "errors and omission." Examples:

> "I'm just a hospital employee. The hospital pays me by the word, and they get what they pay for. Malpractice insurance is their problem, not mine."

> "It's a doctor thing. They dictate it; and they're responsible for checking it. If something's wrong, it's their fault."

> "I don't treat patients. How can I be responsible for someone receiving bad care?"

> "No insurance company offers this type of insurance to medical transcriptionists, and the government says we're just medical secretaries. If I'm just a medical secretary and can't buy insurance for anything else, how can I be liable?"

Why do I believe that medical transcriptionists are likely candidates for professional malpractice exposure and, therefore, purchasers of "errors and omissions" professional liability insurance?

- You have been for years. If you breach the confidentiality of privileged patient records, you are responsible—are you not? This is just another way of saying "doing something that another had a legal right to depend on your not doing" = *error.*

- Historically, most professions evolve into (1) recognition, (2) status, and (3) professional liability. Professional healers were not always physicians; remember barbers and bloodletting?

- Economic forces are creating greater pressures for diversified sources of liability funding. Hospitals, accustomed to physicians, registered nurses, and others having their own professional liability coverage, are seeking to further minimize exposure and decrease insurance costs.

- The system is changing. The hospital has been at the center of health care for several decades. What many take for granted, few remember as different.

- If a facility terminates your employment because you have been accused of wrongdoing, you would no longer be covered under the facility's employee coverage.

It was not until the post World War II boom in demand and growth in public funding that hospitals were perceived as the lodestar of health care. This, in turn, was boosted by the onset of Medicare in the 1960s. Since the early 1980s and the 1992 presidential campaign, however, health care has been diversifying back into the communities and into a patient-centric system.

Hospital-based transcription departments are going to have to justify their existence in quality and economic terms. These terms will increasingly include cost and liability containment. Plus, they are going to have to offer relationships that fit easily into a client's management span of control.

The final point begs some debate: the role and impact of plaintiffs' attorneys in creating the demand for medical transcriptionist liability insurance.

A plaintiff's personal injury/malpractice attorney may sue everybody involved with a patient's case, and sooner or later an attorney will sue a transcriptionist or a service directly. That's the rub; should you have insurance to protect you or should you not have insurance, theorizing that with no insurance money available you will not be an attractive target? It is an illusory choice.

Unless you have taken and are living a vow of poverty, you need "errors and omissions" insurance. Whether hospital-based or independent, employee or employer, this form of business insurance is a cost of doing business.

Reprinted from "Legal Briefs," JAAMT, Vol. 12, No. 6, November-December 1993, pp. 20–21. Copyright AAMT, 1993, Modesto, CA.

Appendix L

Medical Transcription as Communication

Claudia Tessier, CAE, CMT, RRA

Whenever I do medical transcription workshops, I find myself talking about medical transcription as communication. This surprises some MTs until we talk about it more, and then they find that this new perspective helps them to prepare better transcripts.

Think about it. What is the purpose of the transcripts we prepare? Your immediate answer is probably documentation of patient care, and you are right. But take it a step further. For the documentation to be of maximum value, it must communicate the information that the originator wants communicated. That communication serves a variety of purposes: patient care, first and foremost, but also billing, legal, research, and continuing education, to name the most obvious.

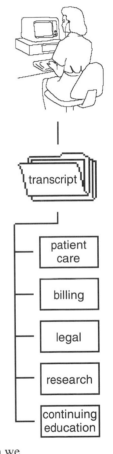

Because the reports we transcribe are communication instruments, they should be complete, consistent, clear, and correct, and they should promote ease of reading. Without these attributes, communication is obstructed. Our goal as medical transcriptionists then is to make our transcripts the best communication instruments we can.

A complete transcript is one that accounts for all the information dictated. In the ideal situation, one in which the dictation is exact and correct in content and form, the transcript would be word for word, with no errors. But let's face it, the ideal situation seldom, if ever, exists. Dictation routinely requires modification as we transform it to the printed word. If we transcribed everything exactly as dictated, we couldn't assure the other attributes (consistency, clarity, and correctness), and we would produce some mighty poor communication instruments. So when we say the transcription is complete, we mean that the report as a whole is complete, that the information dictated is included in the report.

Certainly, to achieve completeness, we must make reasonable efforts not to leave blanks. But sometimes blanks cannot be avoided. The dictation may not be clear (and cannot reasonably be inferred), or new terminology may be used that our research does not uncover, or we may have mechanical difficulties that preclude transcription. When we must leave blanks, we draw them to the attention of the appropriate individual(s), most likely our supervisor and/or the dictating physician. it

So, sometimes, meeting our obligation to provide complete reports means document-ing why they are not complete.

Completeness also requires recording negative and normal results as dictated. Some of you may still be making the beginner's error of deleting such findings. Negative or normal findings, e.g., "normal pelvic exam" or "negative chest x-ray" are significant information. They document that the referenced exam or laboratory work was done, thereby guarding against repetition of the same exam or lab work (and charges for same); in turn this could influence the patient's perception of the care s/he is given, and it could help to control expenses. They may be significant in defending a malpractice suit by providing evidence that the usual level of care was delivered. Negative or normal findings may help to rule in or rule out certain diseases or conditions. They may influence the decision to do further tests or to use certain treatment modalities, including surgery. So don't make the mistake of think-ing they are insignificant because they are negative or normal. The physician is dictating these findings for a reason, and we have the obligation to transcribe them.

We make our transcripts consistent when we stay alert to the meaning and con-text of the dictation so that we recognize inconsistent data and correct it if possible. Sometimes the context of the report permits easy correction. When the physician dictates a hysterectomy on a 45-year-old male, we don't have to think twice about changing it to a 45-year-old female. When the surgeon starts a dictation on a left cataract, then later in the report refers to a right cataract, we probably can't determine which is correct unless we have access to the medical record; so, we leave blanks and draw them to the attention of our supervisor or the dictating physician.

We also make our transcripts consistent by applying standards of transcription practices. AAMT guides us in this regard through its publications and education programs; in particular *Style Guide for Medical Transcription* and the "SOS" column in *JAAMT*.

We seek to achieve clarity in our transcripts when we edit rambling dictation; for example, when the physician dictates a surgical report in one long sentence, we mark the logical breaks through the formation of multiple sentences with appropriate punc-tuation. When misplaced modifiers are dictated, we rephrase the sentence to place them appropriately. When the physical exam is dictated in the history of present illness, we separate it and put it in its own section.

We correct obvious dictation errors and draw attention to those we recognize as errors but don't know how to correct. We recognize punctuation errors and correct them. We silently thank the dictator for spelling a patient's name or a term that s/he thinks we will not recognize, and then we take care to be sure that the patient's name is spelled correctly, and we spell medical terms as we know they should be spelled (*diverticula,* not *diverticuli*) or as our research tells us they should be spelled. We recognize when the wrong word is dictated and make the correction (*mitigate,* not *militate*; *regimen,* not *regime*).

We promote the readability of the report by thinking about how the transcribed words will appear to the reader. We avoid hyphenation at the end of the line because will slow the reader down. Conversely, we use hyphenation when words or word parts, if joined, could easily be misread by the reader, e.g., co-workers instead of coworkers (cow-workers? thinks the reader). We reserve capitalization for required use, recognizing that its overuse diminishes its value and impact. We use abbreviations when we are confident that they can be understood by the reader—and only when dictated—or implied, as is the case with abbreviations for measurement.

We also promote readability through format and organization. Headings and subheadings draw the eye of the reader to the report's major sections and subsections. By transcribing content in its appropriate section (even when not so dictated), we diminish the likelihood of information being missed.

I have given limited examples of how medical transcriptionists play an important role in assuring that the reports we prepare are valuable communication instruments. We quickly recognized that we are medical language specialists. But our role doesn't stop there. We are also communicators, more specifically medical communicators.

Think about that role each time you prepare a transcript. Ask yourself: Do my transcripts communicate complete, consistent, clear, and correct information? Do I prepare them in a manner that enhances their readability? If either or both answers are no, you have identified an important continuing education goal for yourself. Be the best medical communicator you can be.

MTs: Partners in Medical Communication

The partnership begins ...

Medical transcription (the recording of medical treatment and procedures in pictorial or written form) has existed since the beginning of medical care and research.

Ancient cave writings attest to the earliest forms of patient care documentation. While the medium changed from metal plates to clay tablets, to hieroglyphs on temple walls, to papyrus, to parchment, to paper, and most recently to computer, the reasons for maintaining records have always been the same—to record patient care and the achievements in medical science.

Until the twentieth century, physicians served as both providers of medical care and scribes for the medical community. After 1900, when standardization of medical data became critical to research, medical stenographers replaced physicians as scribes, taking their dictation in shorthand.

The advent of dictating equipment made it unnecessary for physician and scribe to work face-to-face, and the career of medical transcription came into being. As physicians came to rely on the judgment and reasoning of experienced medical transcriptionists to safeguard the accuracy and integrity of medical dictation, medical transcription evolved into a medical language specialty. It is now one of the most sophisticated of the allied health professions, creating an important partnership between healthcare providers and those who document patient records.

Medical transcriptionists as professionals

Since 1978, medical transcriptionists have been represented by a professional organization, the American Association for Medical Transcription (AAMT), which has developed a competency profile (COMPRO®) and a model curriculum for transcription educators, as well as a model job description.

AAMT emphasizes continuing education for its members, holding annual conferences for transcriptionists, educators, supervisors and managers, and business owners. There are over 170 local and state/regional AAMT component associations, each of which holds regular educational meetings and symposia.

It is through the efforts of AAMT that medical transcriptionists have become recognized as healthcare professionals with expertise in medical language.

Medical transcription—a medical language specialty

In the broadest sense, medical transcription is the act of translating from oral to printed form (on paper or on computer) the record of a patient's medical history and treatment.

The healthcare industry is moving to create computerized patient records, allowing storage of an individual's entire medical treatment history in one continuous record that can be accessed by physicians and healthcare institutions anywhere.

Physicians and other healthcare providers employ state-of-the-art electronic transmission methods to dictate highly technical information summarizing medical histories, diagnoses, and treatments for their patients. These medical professionals rely on skilled medical transcriptionists to transform spoken words into comprehensive records that accurately communicate medical information.

Keyboarding and transcription should not be confused. The primary skills necessary for performance of quality medical transcription are extensive medical knowledge and understanding, sound judgment, deductive reasoning, and the ability to detect medical inconsistencies in dictation. For example, a diagnosis inconsistent with the patient's history and symptoms may be mistakenly dictated. The medical transcriptionist questions, seeks clarification, verifies the information, and enters it into the report.

Medical transcription is a medical language specialty, a distinction that has led to an alternative title for the qualified medical transcriptionist—*medical language specialist.*

What does a medical language specialist need to know?

Medical transcription requires a practical knowledge of medical terminology, anatomy, physiology, disease processes, and the internal organization of medical reports. A medical language specialist must be aware of standards and requirements that apply to the medical record, as well as the legal significance of medical transcripts.

Medical reports take many forms, including histories and physical examinations, progress reports, emergency room notes, consultations, operative reports, discharge summaries, clinic notes, referral letters, radiology reports, pathology reports, and an array of documentation spanning more than 60 medical specialties and subspecialties! Thus, the medical transcriptionist, or medical language specialist, must be well versed in the language of medicine and surgery.

To prepare for this profession, medical transcriptionists study:

- medical terminology, including Greek and Latin suffixes, prefixes, and roots
- biological science, including anatomy and physiology of all body systems, and various disease processes

- medical science
- medical and surgical procedures, involving thousands of instruments, supplies, appliances, and prosthetic devices
- laboratory values, correlating laboratory test results with patient diagnosis and treatment
- use of medical reference materials and research techniques

What other skills are required to perform medical transcription?

Medical understanding is critical for the professional medical language specialist. The multisyllabic and homonymous terms used in medicine are unlike the language of any other profession.

Quality medical transcription also requires:

- above-average knowledge of English punctuation and grammar
- excellent auditory skills, allowing the transcriptionist to interpret sounds almost simultaneously with keyboarding
- advanced proofreading and editing skills, ensuring accuracy of transcribed material
- versatility in use of transcription equipment and computers, since transcriptionists may work in a variety of settings
- highly developed analytical skills, employing deductive reasoning to convert sounds into meaningful form

What are the characteristics of a medical language specialist?

Medical transcription professionals are:

- word specialists
- self-starters
- perfectionists
- independent by nature
- self-disciplined
- interested in medicine
- committed to learning
- known to have inquiring minds
- able to concentrate for long periods
- willing to assist others
- able to work with minimal supervision
- dedicated to professional development and achievement

Finally, it should be clear that all medical language specialists share a common trait—enthusiasm for their profession.

As one medical transcriptionist puts it, "I love what I do. I work next to a registered nurse turned transcriptionist, a science teacher working part-time in the field, and a biologist. I learn new terms every day, and I am never bored. My fellow medical transcriptionists are intelligent and interesting."

Medical language specialists work together, partnering to build their medical language skills.

Why haven't I heard about medical transcription before?

While medical transcription is among the most fascinating of allied health professions, the general public knows little about those who practice this skill. Transcriptionists have been misclassified as *typists, medical word processors, medical secretaries,* and *dictating machine operators.*

Through the efforts of the American Association for Medical Transcription (AAMT), visibility and recognition of the profession have increased, and the terms *medical transcriptionist* and *medical language specialist* have gained widespread acceptance.

The medical language specialist works in an office setting, usually far removed from the examining rooms, clinics, and hospital wards where patient care is rendered. Patients rarely have the opportunity to hear about those who transcribe their medical reports.

All healthcare providers rely to some extent on the skills of the medical transcriptionist to provide written documentation of patient care. The reports produced by the qualified medical language specialist are the repository of information concerning medical practice. These reports function as legal documentation and fulfill requirements for insurance reimbursement. They also serve as references for scientific research.

Since medical language specialists work in the shadow of the healthcare providers who author and sign medical reports, their partnership role in producing accurate medical records may be indicated only by their initials at the end of a report, alongside those of the dictator.

Where are medical transcriptionists employed?

Medical transcriptionists utilize their talents in a variety of healthcare settings, including doctors' offices, public and private hospitals, teaching hospitals, medical transcription services, clinics, laboratories, radiology and pathology departments, insurance companies, medical libraries, government medical facilities, rehabilitation centers, legal offices, research centers, veterinary medical facilities, and associations representing the healthcare industry.

Medical language specialists work with physicians and surgeons in multiple specialties. They work with pharmacists, therapists, technicians, nurses, dieticians, social workers, psychologists, and other medical personnel. All of these healthcare providers rely on information that is received, documented, and disseminated by the medical language specialist.

Some transcriptionists choose to work out of their homes as employees of transcription services or hospitals. Still others provide services as independent contractors.

Qualified medical transcriptionists who wish to expand their professional responsibilities may choose to become department heads, supervisors, managers, or owners of medical transcription services.

Experienced medical language specialists may become teachers, working in schools and colleges and educating future medical transcriptionists.

Is medical transcription a good home-based business?

Many popular publications sing the praises of medical transcription as a home business, citing the potential for high income with little investment. Courses in medical transcription are proliferating, some offering "quick fixes" for students interested in becoming business owners.

Failure to make the investment in quality education can result not only in business failure but also in shoddy documentation for the real client—the patient.

Medical transcription is a medical language specialty. Fluency in this language is not accomplished merely by completing a basic terminology course and installing a spellchecker in a computer!

The transcriptionist working from home must make a significant investment in equipment and reference material and be willing to make frequent updates to both equipment and library in order to keep up with rapidly changing technology and terminology.

Careful planning and the advice of legal and financial experts are essential to the success of a home-based business.

AAMT advises that the individual considering a home-based medical transcription business first gain experience in a healthcare facility or transcription service under the direction of experienced and qualified medical language specialists.

What makes medical transcription an attractive career choice?

Medical transcription provides unlimited intellectual challenge and the opportunity to make a unique contribution to quality patient care and service.

Healthcare is a rapidly growing field, and the demand for quality documentation is increasing. The profession provides a high level of job security, and skilled medical language specialists may receive a premium for their services.

Because their services are in demand, transcriptionists are often able to arrange convenient and flexible work schedules.

Medical transcription is a portable skill that allows for professional and geographic mobility.

Age restrictions are seldom found, with great value being placed on the experience and knowledge of the mature transcriptionist.

Medical transcription can be a lifelong, satisfying career, providing the constant challenge of an expanding and advancing technology. The changes occurring in the healthcare industry promise to provide even more challenges to the forward-looking medical language specialist.

◆

To learn more about the medical transcription profession and the education and training required to become a partner in medical communication, contact AAMT.

The Myth of Medical Transcription

Pat Forbis, CMT

Webster's Ninth New Collegiate Dictionary defines *myth* as "a popular belief or tradition that has grown up around something or someone."

The myth of medical transcription is found in the belief some share that the ability to manipulate a keyboard is the primary function of a medical transcriptionist. Mythmakers extend the belief to include that the faster the keyboardist, the better the medical transcriptionist.

Is a medical transcriptionist without a keyboard a medical transcriptionist?

By acknowledging that a keyboard is essential to being a medical transcriptionist, are we perpetuating this myth? Is the keyboard an essential factor in the growth and development of the person using it?

Dispelling myths begins with a reality check. Such a reality check was included in AAMT's 1981 annual meeting slogan, "The Mind Behind the Machine." The "AAMT Model Job Description: Medical Transcriptionist" and this year's National Medical Transcriptionist Week theme, "Medical Transcriptionists: The Medical Language Specialists," boldly announce that it's time to recognize that a medical transcriptionist's primary attribute is not in the fingertips.

If we believe that mind over keyboard is the main ingredient of the medical transcriptionist, we need to think about how far we can venture from the keyboard and still refer to ourselves as medical transcriptionists.

My introduction to medical transcription was no different than that of most people in my age group. My on-the-job indoctrination was keyboard oriented, and my prime time was absorbed with "do it faster, faster, faster." The keyboard became my hamster wheel. I fell in step with the furry little creatures, running with my fingers at top speed up and down, back and forth, until I could type not one more keystroke. Stopping to catch my breath and give my fingers, arms, and neck a rest, I would take stock of my production. Funny how the week's average would not change much. But, if it fell below my production expectations, I was stressed because I felt I had let myself down. The quality of my work was never an issue because no one ever reviewed it.

It wasn't until I started proofreading others' work that I realized I was a participant in the myth of medical transcription. My attention had been focused on keyboarding skills, not on my fund of knowledge. It was time to turn on the power switch to my mind. How much was there to learn? What I had considered to be a profession with limited opportunity now appeared to have limitless possibilities. In order to arrive at that conclusion I had to do what the 1981 slogan suggested and move my mind behind the machine. In so doing I was able to recognize that not all available career opportunities were dependent upon the keyboard.

Must medical transcriptionists change careers in order to achieve professional growth? No, because we've confirmed that being a medical transcriptionist is not synonymous with keyboard productivity. In the climate of change we are experiencing, medical transcriptionists can be practitioners with minimal or no keyboard-generated production. When climates change, it is important to pay attention and remain alert. What might fall from the sky or wash ashore could be significant to our future.

If we analyze what knowledge medical transcriptionists share, we find strengths in languages (English and medicine), reasoning and editing skills, proofreading, and keyboarding. Many transcriptionists have become knowledgeable in software, hardware, and computer applications. And, although the majority of transcriptionists have not been instructors in a classroom setting, most have been educators by sharing their important knowledge with struggling novices. Management and supervisory training has placed medical transcriptionists in decision-making positions. Professional development and business courses have paved the way into the corporate environment.

Just how far does medical transcription reach? The U.S. Department of Labor Statistics tells us that by the year 2000, one of every four workers in the United States will speak English as a second language. Medical transcription has already been identified as a profession suffering from an acute shortage of qualified people; indications are it may get worse.

We won't need to go far from the keyboard to utilize our medical knowledge. Consider the following:

- Coders are in demand. Coding is also a medical language speciality. Medical transcriptionists have participated in coding with relative ease because of their existing knowledge of medicine.

- Medical transcription educators are being recruited in a variety of settings: court reporting schools, junior colleges, proprietary schools, and vo-tech programs. Educators are even being recruited for off-shore programs. Hospital education departments, insurance companies, and others in need of medical terminology call for assistance from those who speak the language.

- Authoring and editing are possibilities. Reference materials are always in short supply. Not all specialties have word books, and in the constantly changing world of medicine, the need for revisions in existing materials is never ending.

Pharmaceutical companies, researchers, and technical manual developers are among those who need the medical transcriptionist's expertise.

• Consulting can be done for hospitals who employ medical transcriptionists or for start-up transcription services, for software companies who are developing medical dictionaries and word lists, or for educational administrators who want to implement transcription programs.

• Medical transcriptionists can be quality assurance experts, department heads, managers. Who is more qualified to supervise the preparation of or critique medical documentation than a medical transcriptionist?

• And in AAMT's office: positions such as medical transcriptionist or education services coordinator offer other exciting alternatives. Who better than qualified medical transcriptionists can oversee these important functions?

All of these opportunities require the knowledge the medical transcriptionist possesses. Productivity of a different kind is required. Does that mean the individuals who meet these challenges are not medical transcriptionists? I think not.

It is said that if something is repeated for 21 consecutive days it becomes a habit. Habits are formed with relative ease; breaking habits is not done overnight. Breaking the keyboard productivity habit is a process of withdrawal and rehabilitation. Like eliminating any habit, one must exercise self-discipline and determination. Certainly it takes more than three weeks of practice to make such a transition. Risk is involved. Not only must you think differently, you must perform differently. There are shifts in responsibilities, personal expectations, and what is expected of you. It is important to set aside the keyboard-generated productivity habits in order to think about these new challenges and contemplate the risks. What if I can't ... what if it's too ... what if it doesn't... on and on.

Physical relocation as well as mental relocation may be necessary. Physical relocation can also be risky. New environments mean uprooting and upheaval: meeting new people, finding a new place to live, leaving friends and family. It is important to have a clear understanding of your individual goals and career expectations when breaking old habits and making new ones of this magnitude.

Arriving at the decision to make changes marks the beginning of an exciting adventure. It reminds me of drag racing (something I've always loved to do) when you've taken the car as far as you possibly can in first gear so you pop the clutch and hope you don't miss second gear. It's exhilarating when you cross the finish line.

When you view the keyboard as something that is available if you wish to use it and not essential to your performance, but your medical transcriptionist's mind is still consumed with medical transcription research, development, concerns and information, you will be secure in the knowledge that you are a medical transcriptionist, with or without a keyboard.

If you read this column closely, you may wonder: Is there a rite of passage? Can medical transcription supervisors, educators, authors, etc., who have never transcribed be legitimately included in the definition of medical transcriptionists? We'll explore the answer to this question in the next issue of *JAAMT*.

Reprinted from "Impressions," JAAMT, Vol. 10, No. 6, November-December 1991, pp. 6–7. Copyright 1991, AAMT, Modesto, CA.

AAMT Model Job Description: MEDICAL TRANSCRIPTIONIST

The *AAMT Model Job Description* is a practical, useful compilation of the basic job responsibilities of a medical transcriptionist. It is designed to assist human resource managers, department managers, supervisors, and others in recruiting, supervising, and evaluating individuals in medical transcription positions.

The *AAMT Model Job Description* is not intended as a complete list of specific duties and responsibilities. Nor is it intended to limit or modify the right of any supervisor to assign, direct, and control the work of employees under supervision. The use of a particular expression or illustration describing duties shall not be held to exclude other duties not mentioned that are of a similar kind or level of difficulty.

Position Summary: Medical language specialist who interprets and transcribes dictation by physicians and other healthcare professionals regarding patient assessment, workup, therapeutic procedures, clinical course, diagnosis, prognosis, etc., in order to document patient care and facilitate delivery of healthcare services.

Knowledge, skills, and abilities:
1. Minimum education level of associate degree or equivalent in work experience and continuing education.
2. Knowledge of medical terminology, anatomy and physiology, clinical medicine, surgery, diagnostic tests, radiology, pathology, pharmacology, and the various medical specialties as required in areas of responsibility.
3. Knowledge of medical transcription guidelines and practices.
4. Excellent written and oral communication skills, including English usage, grammar, punctuation, and style.
5. Ability to understand diverse accents and dialects and varying dictation styles.
6. Ability to use designated reference materials.
7. Ability to operate designated word processing, dictation, and transcription equipment, and other equipment as specified.
8. Ability to work independently with minimal supervision.
9. Ability to work under pressure with time constraints.
10. Ability to concentrate.
11. Excellent listening skills.
12. Excellent eye, hand, and auditory coordination.
13. Certified medical transcriptionist (CMT) status preferred.

Working conditions:
General office environment. Quiet surroundings. Adequate lighting.

Physical demands:
Primarily sedentary work, with continuous use of earphones, keyboard, foot control, and where applicable, video display terminal.

Job responsibilities:	Performance standards:
1. Transcribes medical dictation to provide a permanent record of patient care.	1.1 Applies knowledge of medical terminology, anatomy and physiology, and English language rules to the transcription and proofreading of medical dictation from originators with various accents, dialects, and dictation styles.
	1.2 Recognizes, interprets, and evaluates inconsistencies, discrepancies, and inaccuracies in medical dictation, and appropriately edits, revises, and clarifies them without altering the meaning of the dictation or changing the dictator's style.
	1.3 Clarifies dictation which is unclear or incomplete, seeking assistance as necessary.
	1.4 Flags reports requiring the attention of the supervisor or dictator.
	1.5 Uses reference materials appropriately and efficiently to facilitate the accuracy, clarity, and completeness of reports.
	1.6 Meets quality and productivity standards and deadlines established by employer.
	1.7 Verifies patient information for accuracy and completeness.
	1.8 Formats reports according to established guidelines.
2. Demonstrates an understanding of the medicolegal implications and responsibilities related to the transcription of patient records to protect the patient and the business/institution.	2.1 Understands and complies with policies and procedures related to medicolegal matters, including confidentiality, amendment of medical records, release of information, patients' rights, medical records as legal evidence, informed consent, etc.

Job responsibilities:	Peformance standards:
	2.2 Meets standards of professional and ethical conduct.
	2.3 Recognizes and reports unusual circumstances and/or information with possible risk factors to appropriate risk management personnel.
	2.4 Recognizes and reports problems, errors, and discrepancies in dictation and patient records to appropriate manager.
	2.5 Consults appropriate personnel regarding dictation which may be regarded as unprofessional, frivolous, insulting, inflammatory, or inappropriate.
3. Operates designated word processing, dictation, and transcription equipment as directed to complete assignments.	3.1 Uses designated equipment effectively, skillfully, and efficiently.
	3.2 Maintains equipment and work area as directed.
	3.3 Assesses condition of equipment and furnishings, and reports need for replacement or repair.
4. Follows policies and procedures to contribute to the efficiency of the medical transcription department.	4.1 Demonstrates an understanding of policies, procedures, and priorities, seeking clarification as needed.
	4.2 Reports to work on time, as scheduled, and is dependable and cooperative.
	4.3 Organizes and prioritizes assigned work, and schedules time to accommodate work demands, turnaround-time requirements, and commitments.
	4.4 Maintains required records, providing reports as scheduled and upon request.
	4.5 Participates in quality assurance programs.
	4.6 Participates in evaluation and selection of equipment and furnishings.
	4.7 Provides administrative/clerical/technical support as needed and as assigned.

Job responsibilities:	Performance standards:
5. Expands job-related knowledge and skills to improve performance and adjust to change.	5.1 Participates in inservice and continuing education activities. 5.2 Provides documentation of inservice and continuing education activities. 5.3 Reviews trends and developments in medicine, English usage, technology, and transcription practices, and shares knowledge with colleagues. 5.4 Documents new and revised terminology, definitions, styles, and practices for reference and application. 5.5 Participates in the evaluation and selection of books, publications, and other reference materials.
6. Uses interpersonal skills effectively to build and maintain cooperative working relationships.	6.1 Works and communicates in a positive and cooperative manner with management and supervisory staff, medical staff, co-workers and other healthcare personnel, and patients and their families when providing information and services, seeking assistance and clarification, and resolving problems. 6.2 Contributes to team efforts. 6.3 Carries out assignments responsibly. 6.4 Participates in a positive and cooperative manner during staff meetings. 6.5 Handles difficult and sensitive situations tactfully. 6.6 Responds well to supervision. 6.7 Shares information with co-workers. 6.8 Assists with training of new employees as needed.

AAMT gratefully acknowledges Lanier Worldwide, Inc., Atlanta, for funding the development of the *AAMT Model Job Description: Medical Transcriptionist.*

For additional information, contact AAMT, P.O. Box 576187, Modesto, CA 95357-6187. Telephone 209-551-0883 or 800-982-2182. Fax 209-551-9317.

Customizing Productivity Standards

Carolyn Wilkinson, CMT

S everal years ago when our medical transcription department decided to develop performance standards, we began by surveying other area hospitals to see what they were doing along these lines. We found that very few had specific standards for quality and quantity, and the standards that did exist didn't apply to us. Our ultimate goal was to establish fair and achievable standards for our employees. We decided everyone would be more satisfied with the results if the standards we developed were based upon the experience and characteristics within our own department.

In the process of developing our standards, we came to several conclusions which kept us true to our goal and which continue to work for us. Listed below are some of those conclusions:

- Performance standards should balance quality and quantity. While timeliness is important, the integrity of a medical document is established by the accuracy of its content, not by the speed with which it is produced.

- Quality assessment should be based upon specific criteria and accepted sources of reference and should always be carried out by medical transcriptionists with extensive knowledge of the work being evaluated.

- The method used to capture and record productivity data should be consistent and completely reliable. The more automated the process, the less likely the results will be questioned.

- Standards should reflect current working conditions and levels of individual ability and should be reviewed periodically to assure continued applicability.

- Performance comparisons among medical transcriptionists from different work environments should be avoided. Significant variances in employee experience and training, the nature and content of dictation, the age and functionality of equipment, and the physical environment in which employees function all have a significant effect on their ability to process information and transcribe it into text.

- Realistic standards take into consideration **all** the factors affecting productivity.

Developing quantity standards

Our first step in developing quantity standards was deciding **what** we were going to count, **how** the counting would be done, and **the format** for recording the resulting data.

The unit of measure we selected was a 60-character line. Our word processing system has a "line count" program which counts keystrokes and converts the total to lines. The line unit is a variable and can be set to individual specifications. Productivity data was recorded on a daily basis for about three months.

We recorded and analyzed the performance of our employees and compared that with what was needed to meet turnaround requirements. In other words, we compared what we had been doing with what we needed to be doing. By using information from our own work setting, employees and managers agreed that our expectations were more likely to be reasonable and appropriate.

We devised a simple formula for determining the average individual productivity rates by dividing the total number of units produced by each transcriptionist by the number of hours that individual worked during the same period. Determining the average hourly productivity rate for the department as a whole was then just a matter of adding together all individual totals and dividing by the total number of hours worked. The same formula was used for both determinations (Example A). Since we already had time records for this period, that part of the information was readily available.

Once individual and department averages had been determined, we were ready to start developing the quantity portion of our standards. Approximately 60% of our employees were functioning at or above the department average; the performance of the remaining 40% was divided between below-average and above-average levels. We decided to set the minimum acceptable level of productivity at 75% of the department average (Example B). We developed an average range of performance by using the minimum standards as the bottom of the range and the department average as the top of the range (Example C).

Developing quality standards

Designing an acceptable method for evaluating quality and accuracy was more complex. We realized that it would be impossible to examine every page of transcription produced in the department, but we needed a sample size that would give a reasonably accurate picture of individual work quality.

Our initial quality analysis plan has been adjusted and fine-tuned over the years and, in its current form, evaluates a full day's work, once a month, for each individual, for a total of 12 samples annually. The samples are randomly selected, varying the primary work assignment and the day of the week.

The method of evaluation is a line-by-line review of each page in the sample. Errors are marked on printed copies of the documents, and an evaluation sheet is filled out for each sample batch. The document copies and evaluation sheet are returned to the transcriptionist, along with comments and suggestions by the transcription supervisor, who conducts the evaluations. The evaluation sheet lists the number of errors in each of six categories, each with a point rating (Example D).

The most difficult part of the process was deciding what we considered a "reasonable" number of errors. What we finally came up with was an error-rating system allowing a maximum number of error points per equivalent page. To balance the variance in page lengths, we developed an "equivalent page" composed of 2,500 characters. We set the maximum acceptable error rate at 1.0 points, or an average of no more than one, 1-point error per equivalent page (Example D).

We developed a separate set of quantity and quality standards for those transcriptionists with less than one year of hospital experience (Medical Transcriptionist I). We felt it was reasonable to expect individuals in this category to be able to meet 50% of the minimum productivity and accuracy standards by the end of six months, and 75% of the minimum standards by the end of nine months. We felt we could expect them to be performing at or above the minimum standard by the end of their first year of employment (Example C).

To encourage improved performance in both quality and quantity, we included an incentive pay program for the Medical Transcriptionist II position as part of the package. To discourage any temptation to sacrifice quality in favor of quantity, we made meeting the minimum standard for quality a prerequisite for participation.

Our efforts to keep pace with changes in technology and activity have necessitated adjustments to the original standards, but we are convinced today that our approach was the right one for our department. The implementation of applicable performance standards has enabled us to be much more objective in evaluating employee performance and in our responses to fluctuations in workload.

For us, individualized standards helped in developing what we—medical transcriptionists and managers—agree is an objective means of evaluating overall performance.

Example A

$$\frac{\text{units produced}}{\text{hours worked}} = \text{hourly productivity rate}$$

Example B

$$\text{department average } (\text{ x }) 75\% = \text{minimum standard}$$

Example C

MEDICAL TRANSCRIPTIONIST I
(less than one year of hospital experience)

3 months

Becoming familiar with equipment, procedures, document format and content; demonstrating progressive improvement in productivity and accuracy.

6 months

Performing at 50% of the minimum standard for productivity and accuracy.

9 months

Performing at 75% of the minimum standard for productivity and accuracy.

12 months

Performing at or above the minimum standard for productivity and accuracy.

MEDICAL TRANSCRIPTIONIST II
(more than one year of hospital experience)

Needs improvement:

Average productivity less than 100% of minimum standard.

Meets the standard:

Average productivity rate between minimum standard and department average.

Exceeds the standard:

Average productivity rate greater than department average.

Example D

$$\frac{\text{number of characters}}{\text{average page size}} = \text{equivalent pages}$$

Example D (continued)

$$\frac{\text{total errors}}{\text{equivalent pages}} = \text{error rate}$$

$$\frac{\text{amount of work evaluated}}{\text{total work performed}} = \text{sample rate}$$

A full-time employee works an average of 20 days each month; one day's work out of every 20 represents a ratio of 1:20, or a 5% sample rate ($1 \div 20 = .05$ or 5%).

QUALITY ANALYSIS WORK SHEET

NAME:_____   DATE PERFORMED:_____

CHARACTER COUNT: (   ) ÷ (2,500) = (   ) EQUIVALENT PAGES

TYPE OF ERROR	RATING		NUMBER OF ERRORS		TOTAL
Medical error	2	x	_____	=	_____
Text omitted	2	x	_____	=	_____
Missing or incorrect patient identification	1	x	_____	=	_____
Spelling, medical	1	x	_____	=	_____
Spelling, nonmedical	1	x	_____	=	_____
Punctuation, grammar or syntax error	0.50	x	_____	=	_____

TOTAL ERRORS . . . . (_____)

$$\frac{\text{TOTAL ERRORS}}{\text{EQUIVALENT PAGES}} = \text{ERROR RATE}$$

Exceeds the standard: 0.00 to 0.40   Meets the standard: 0.50 to 0.99
Needs improvement: 1.0 & above

COMMENTS:

RECOMMENDATIONS:

EVALUATION PERFORMED BY:

Reprinted from JAAMT, Vol. 11, No. 1, January-February 1992, pp. 38–40. Copyright 1992, AAMT, Modesto, CA.

How Much Wood Should a Woodchuck (or a Medical Transcriptionist) **Chuck?**

Pat Forbis, CMT

Woodchucks and medical transcriptionists have a lot of work to do. Remaining focused on the task at hand, working diligently for long periods of time—both make progress. And given just the right amount of quality time, knowledge and experience, both deliver a final product.

How much wood can a woodchuck chuck surely depends on the variables of woodchucking: the kind of wood that is involved, the condition of the woodchuck's teeth, the number of times the woodchuck needs to rest during the day, the interruptions encountered by the woodchuck, and whether the woodchuck is a novice or an old saw, so to speak.

How much work should an average medical transcriptionist (MT) be able to produce during a given period of time? This is the question managers, supervisors, and other statistics gatherers have asked since the bonding between medical language, people, and keyboards. And even though the AAMT model job description provides sound criteria for selecting and evaluating MTs, many who hire transcriptionists and manage transcription environments continue to seek a national average productivity standard. Yet medical transcriptionists also encounter variables ... many variables.

The answer to the question of how much work an average medical transcriptionist should be able to produce comes in two parts: bad news and good news. The bad news is that there is no such thing as a national average productivity standard for medical transcription. The good news is that productivity averages can be determined within individual work settings. The data then can provide assistance for future planning and budgeting.

Preparing medical transcription productivity statistics can be compared to preparing a financial statement. Just as line-item entries must be individually listed in order to determine income and expense, medical transcription variables must be taken into consideration before accurate productivity can be determined. Substitute income and expense variables with transcription input and output variables in order to prepare the productivity statement.

In the final analysis, the productivity statement is exactly like a financial statement. It is a "snapshot" of the moment in time which the statement was prepared and reflects the historical events (variables) leading to the bottom line (average productivity for the period of time examined).

Careful review or audit of financial data can be helpful in budget preparation and determination of future needs. Analysis of productivity statements can be helpful in determining medical transcription needs and expectations, as well as diminishing frustration of managers and supervisors whose knowledge of medical transcription may be limited. Analysis of productivity standards can also assist in setting goals and projections.

Here are some line items that are medical transcription variables (with examples):

Input

- **Dictator characteristics** (English as a first or second language, voice characteristics, articulation skills, new or experienced dictator)
- **Dictation equipment characteristics** (analog, digital, controls, maintenance, media quality)
- **Type of report** (operative, discharge, progress notes, H&P, radiology, pathology, specialty)
- **Completeness of dictation** (provision of patient demographics, use of abbreviations, incomplete reports)
- **Difficulty factors of reports** (routine or complex; new procedures, drugs, instruments)
- **Environmental factors** (background noise, sound quality)

Output

- **MT knowledge** (education, experience, language, fluency, familiarity with types of reports, familiarity with dictating staff)
- **MT equipment awareness** (experience on facility equipment, including keyboard, hardware, software, printers or modems, macros, formats, dictionaries)
- **Transcription equipment characteristics** (quality, features, maintenance)
- **Resource availability** (adequate, up-to-date, accessible references; access to other MTs)
- **Environmental factors** (ergonomics, distractions)
- **Performance expectations** (demands for quantity, demands for quality, personnel policies)
- **Other responsibilities** (answering telephone, filing, assisting other MTs)

The historical performance of an individual medical transcriptionist or an entire department can be determined by establishing the method to quantify productivity and then tracking productivity over a period of time. If all factors remain the same, future productivity can be expected to remain the same. However, if one or more input or output factors change, average productivity (individual and collective) will change. In other words, if the same transcriptionists work at the same equipment and interpret the same dictators, who use no new drugs, instruments, procedures, etc., the productivity statement should remain the same. Something as simple as a new chair, however, can alter productivity.

Productivity data can be helpful in transcription process analysis and needs assessment. If there are significant differences in MT productivity, the output variables will provide valuable information. If transcriptionist *A* produces 500 lines a day (a line is anything you want it to be) and transcriptionist *B* produces 2,000 a day, one should ask why there is a significant difference and what can be done to stabilize it.

Ask some questions:

• Does *A* need to work on skill building?
  If so, are in service programs available to assist the individual?

• Does *B* produce 2,000 lines of quality transcription?
  The definition of quality is not quantity. Peer review or quality assurance should be practiced in all transcription environments.

• Does *A* have responsibilities other than transcription?
  A may be answering the phones, looking for reports, etc. Transcription productivity will be influenced by ancillary responsibility.

• Does *A* speak the language of medicine as fluently as *B?*
  Transcription is a language specialty. Just as one learns fluency in Spanish, French, or other foreign language, the medical language must be integrated into one's thought processes before it can be utilized effectively. Continuing education for MTs is essential.

• Does *B* use appropriate shortcuts that drive productivity upward?
  Software packages are available that use "tekkie shorthand" which enables skilled users to boost productivity considerably.

• Do *A* and *B* have equal reference materials?
  Adequate reference materials are essential in preparing accurate reports. Sharing references can slow productivity.

• Does *B* willingly assist other MTs who have questions?
  If productivity demands are high, some MTs will insist on isolation.

Equipment failures, lighting, furniture, poor dictating habits, inadequate breaks, ringing telephones or other noise, clerical assignments such as copying, filing, or delivering work ... many factors contribute to variations in productivity.

Yet the search will continue for the average medical transcriptionist. She or he will be lurking behind an average computer screen somewhere in an average transcription environment in an average medical facility or office in an average community.

Language skills, medical knowledge, and keyboarding coordination will be average, and she or he will be privileged to receive average dictation from average dictators who perform average procedures on average patients. The difficulty level of the report will be average, and the report will be dictated on average equipment at an average rate and volume in an average dialect.

This individual will have access to an average reference library, and his/her ergonomic surroundings will contain a chair of average height at an average desk in average lighting. Management expectations will be average, as will be format design and quality/quantity demands.

One thing can be said for certain about the average day of both the woodchuck and the medical transcriptionist; it's unlike any other known to man or woman.

Reprinted with permission from "AAMT Track," ADVANCE, October 12, 1992.

Appendix R

The Q-P Zone

Terri Wakefield, CMT

The discussion related to quality and productivity standards in medical transcription is a recurring one. As cost-conscious healthcare employers recognize the necessity to ensure the quality of care at the least possible cost to the patient, employees are feeling the effects of this through more stringent work standards. This is especially recognized in medical transcription departments.

So, let's come up with a national standard for medical transcription productivity. It would be nice if there were such an animal, wouldn't it? Employers/managers/supervisors would be able to do their jobs much more quickly and efficiently if someone would just do the difficult and time-consuming task of developing a productivity standard for them. Alas, the expectation is unrealistic, and we must meet this two-headed monster straight on!

Can AAMT—or anyone else for that matter—in fairness to all transcriptionists and their employers and supervisors, provide a valid national productivity standard? I think not. Though a national standard based on certain criteria could be a guide, it would inevitably lead to concrete decisions with little regard to the differences in work settings. It is foreseeable that facilities would hear or read about a national standard and implement it without the accompanying admonishment to use it as a guide to establishing a workable standard for that particular facility.

Case in point

If an MT worked in a 600-bed teaching hospital, transcribed dictation from over 300 physicians, pulled charts, copied reports, answered the telephone, helped other transcriptionists, etc., that MT would be unhappy if the supervisor required a standard of "x" hundred lines (of "x" length) a day based on the fact that it was a national standard.

On the other hand, if an MT worked in a transcription service, transcribing material from a select group of dictators, with a clerk that did the retrieval and copying, had a well-lit station with an ergonomically fitted chair, and used state-of-the-art equipment,"x" lines a day might not be an unfair standard. But—I say **might** not be. It is important to recognize there are so many variables, even these scenarios cannot provide all the information that will ultimately determine an appropriate productivity standard for a particular setting.

You are now entering the Q-P zone: proceed with caution

The emphasis has been on a productivity standard, but this gives a distorted view. Let's not forget that QUALITY must be the first priority. Quality and productivity together (hence the "Q-P Zone") must be considered as ONE standard, not individual entities. When developing the "standard," emphasis must be placed on allowing quality and productivity to complement each other for the efficient and accurate transcription of medical documents.

Medical transcriptionists are professionals. They recognize the importance of quality in their work; they recognize the importance of transcribing the dictation in a timely manner.

In search of a national standard

Okay, it's established that a medical transcription productivity standard cannot be set that will fit everyone's circumstances. Now what?

AAMT **does** recommend certain medical transcription standards. *The Style Guide for Medical Transcription* provides style and practice standards for medical transcription. This journal has a continuing column on standards ("SOS: Standards of Style"). With the input of thousands of expert transcriptionists across the country, who is better qualified than AAMT to provide these standards? There are excellent resources in medical dictionaries, word books, text books, etc., to provide standards for the appropriate use of medical terms. Individual facilities often provide required formats, stylistic preferences, and standards for the transcription of medical reports.

When conflicts occur, the MTs with their supervisor/managers must then make an educated judgment on what will be the standard for that situation.

When quality standards, including style, medical terms, formats, etc., are in place, productivity is enhanced. MTs need not repeatedly search references or ask how certain material should be transcribed.

Common units of measure include lines, minutes of dictation, keystrokes, and characters. Each includes variables that have to be defined. If lines are counted, factors to be determined include length of the line, how carriage returns are counted, how half lines are dealt with, etc. Using minutes of dictation, one has to take into account the vast differences in physicians' rates of dictation.

The most efficient unit of productivity measure in medical transcription is the character. For the sake of discussion, in this article we are considering the character as the "output character" or the actual characters that are in the final document. It is, of course, possible to count "input" characters (keystrokes) as some equipment can count this for you. If you use machine-counted characters, are glossaries/macros being used? This, of course, results in fewer keystrokes input and more characters output on the final document. Is the equipment counting all function keys, corrections, etc.?

Quality is measured on the final document, not on how someone inputs the information. To establish a quality/productivity standard, the standard should be based on the same measurement medium—the final document.

There are many variables to consider when developing a productivity/quality standard and why one standard does not fit all. For example: Experience/expertise of the transcriptionist. Teaching facilities vs small rural hospitals. Number of different dictators and types of procedures. The quality of the dictation. The accent/dialect of the dictator. Transcriptionists who do repetitive reports vs a variety of procedures. Simple reports vs complex reports. Equipment used: keyboards, dictation equipment, transcribers, tapes. Non-transcription work that is required (phone, training, questions, copying, retrieving charts, delivering reports). Availability of current reference materials. Etc., etc., etc. Only the individual facility can determine the variables pertinent to that facility and develop a Q-P standard that takes those variables into accounts.

In the fall 1987 and winter 1987–1988 issues of *JAAMT,* there were two articles written on quality and productivity standards ("Work Standards You Can Live With, Part I: Quantity Standards" and "Work Standards You Can Live With, Part II: Quality Standards" by Marilyn Craddock, CMT, RRA). These articles provide important insights into the development of quality and productivity standards for medical transcription. The author recognized that the development of these standards needs to emphasize the work environment. A department self-study is suggested to define what the quality and productivity have been for that setting, and then a basis is established for developing the standards, again for that setting. In this way, the standard (quality and productivity) is developed based on the specific circumstances of the individual facility's work environment—not on someone else's!

Communicating the unknown

When it is recognized that a quality and productivity standard must be implemented, the medical transcriptionists should be involved in the process. MTs have an integral knowledge of what is going on around them, what is affecting quality and productivity, and they can give valuable input in developing the standard.

Most transcriptionists would welcome a fair and equitable standard: one that reflects professionalism, the particular work environment and characteristics, and expertise. Developing a standard and then trying to implement it without having the input from the people it is going to affect most is a grave error. Not only will morale suffer, but quality and productivity—the very goals sought—will suffer.

MTs can help develop a quality program through suggestions and inservice programs with discussions on appropriate transcription practices, acceptable alternatives, and problem areas. Positive communication between MTs and supervisors/managers is essential when decisions have to be made that will affect a work standard.

Set mutual goals

Implementing a new standard or making needed changes in an established standard takes time. The time required to make changes will depend on the extent of those changes. If the transcription department has never had a quality control program, some MTs may have acquired bad habits and inconsistencies that have never been brought to their attention. If the supervisor is a non-MT, s/he must become knowledgeable about medical transcription and aware of the characteristics particular to that department and institution.

The requirement that changes be made overnight in the quality of transcription is unrealistic and unnecessary. Transcriptionists and their supervisors should work together to set fair and mutually agreed upon goals. Issues can be addressed in inservice or group discussions, and reasonable time lines set for the transcriptionists to make needed changes.

Providing continuing education opportunities on a regular basis will enhance the quality and productivity of the medical transcriptionists. This might be accomplished through participation in a local chapter of AAMT. Also, MTs can attend continuing education programs, inservices, grand rounds, etc., provided to nurses, doctors, and other staff at local hospitals.

The solution

The search for a one-size-fits-all quality and productivity standard will probably continue for a long time. There are no easy answers, but there are suggestions on making the process easier and yet tailored to the specific transcription site. AAMT provides a recommended unit of measure and provides standards for practice and style. Quality and productivity articles have been written to help establish guidelines.

Although the process may take some time, the end result will be a standard for quality and productivity that will be efficient for the employer as well as the medical transcriptionist.

They're Asking the Wrong Questions

Claudia Tessier, CAE, CMT, RRA

O ne of the most common questions we in the AAMT office hear is "What is the national productivity standard for medical transcription?" or its variants "How many lines should I expect my MTs to transcribe per day?" and "What does the average MT produce in a day?" These questions frequently come from non-MTs who are supervising or managing medical transcription departments or services. It seems that the less the inquirers know about medical transcription, the more insistent they are that there must be a national standard—and if there isn't, there certainly should be!

When we reply that the only reasonable productivity standard for their work environment is the one they establish and periodically revise based on the unique characteristics of their dictation, dictators, equipment, MTs, MT job descriptions, patient mix, types of reports, etc., they first express frustration, then they ask for help.

As we guide them toward establishing a reasonable standard based on their own characteristics, we encourage them to give even more attention to the quality of the transcription. Some have difficulty with this. If medical transcription is supervised by those naive enough to think some magical national figure will determine the appropriate productivity level for their department, it is not surprising that they have not addressed the quality of that same medical transcription.

But before they can adequately do their job, they are going to have to recognize and accept that a lot of bad medical transcription will never make up for a smaller quantity of good transcription.

But what is good transcription? To answer that question, you must know how to distinguish what is accurate from what isn't. You must know the answer to the fundamental question: What is an error?

Well, errors come in a variety of shapes and sizes. Some of the more common shapes are:

- Typographical error—*hte.*

- Spelling error—*accomodation.*

- Wrong word—*installation* instead of *instillation.*

- Punctuation error—*She was to return in one week, however, her condition worsened and she was seen in the emergency room eight hours later.*

- Grammatical error—*Neither pain nor guarding were present.*

- Leaving a blank when the dictation is clear and the MT should be expected to know the term.

- Guessing instead of leaving a blank when the dictation is not clear and it would be unreasonable to expect the MT to know the term or phrase.

- Transcribing as dictated when it is reasonable to expect the MT to recognize that the dictation is inaccurate—*The incision was made in the left eye. ... After removing the cataract from the right eye, we closed the incision ...*

- Inappropriate editing, when the MT edits unnecessarily or in a manner that changes the meaning or significantly alters the dictator's style.

- Format error, for example, when the physician dictates allergies within the social history and the MT does not edit appropriately.

- Physician's spelling error that the MT transcribes as dictated—*diverticuli* for *diverticula.*

- Proofreading error, for example, when the MT relies on the spellchecker for proofreading and it doesn't recognize that a correctly spelled word is the wrong word—*enema* for *intima.*

- Inconsistency—*This 45-year-old male is status post hysterectomy.*

- Made-up term—*rambid* for *rapid.*

- Nonsense term—*papal edema* for *papilledema.*

- Missing transcription, for example, when the MT doesn't transcribe the dictation completely and doesn't leave a blank to indicate that it is incomplete.

- Inaccurate presentation of lab data—*pH 741.*

- Wrong hyphenation—*cholecystect-omy.*

- Wrong presentation of term—*KCL* for *KCl.*

- Wrong word—*Lanoxin* for *digoxin.*

- Wrong numeric value—*Valium 50 mg* instead of *5 mg.*

As for error size, they come in small and large: Small ones don't change the meaning of the report. Most are typographical errors or grammatical errors, but you will find some spelling errors here too.

Large errors influence meaning and are most likely to include wrong words, inaccurate presentation of lab data, guessing, wrong doses, some spelling errors. It isn't always the "shape" or type of error that determines its size. Rather it is the context of the report, i.e., the impact of the error on the meaning of the report.

It isn't always easy to recognize errors. Measuring quality requires higher level skills and more knowledge than measuring quantity. But until those responsible for evaluating MTs recognize that quality is more important than quantity, neither the patient nor the dictating physician nor the institution nor the medical transcriptionist—not even the supervisor or manager—will be served adequately and fairly.

To evaluate medical transcriptionists, evaluators must be able to evaluate medical transcription. Evaluators must be able to answer the questions "What is correct?" and "What is an error?" If the evaluators can't answer those questions, it doesn't matter whether they can measure quantity.

Reprinted from JAAMT, *Vol. 10, No. 4, July-August 1991, p. 2. Copyright 1991, AAMT, Modesto, CA.*

Appendix T

Transcription by the Pound

Pat Forbis, CMT

Technology has evolutionized and revolutionized communication and information throughout the world. Early predictions regarding voice recognition technology caused us to consider our professional mortality. Computerization, we were told, would become such a routine way of life that not only would we be relieved of the functional duties of daily living, our need to speak to one another would be minimal to nonexistent. When we did find it necessary to communicate, computerese would be the vocabulary of choice. Instead of replacement, however, we witnessed rethinking, redoing, and many new professional opportunities.

Although technology has done wonderful things for the medical transcriptionist, it is also responsible for fanning the flame of serious number crunchers. There is a place for number crunchers, even in medical transcription. But, the good they do is intermingled with some notions that appear to be noble but are hard to legitimize.

For example, the request from supervisors and managers for average productivity standards has strummed many number crunchers' entrepreneurial chords. These self-proclaimed experts have a one-size-fits-all remedy for supervisors, managers, administrators, and anyone else who wants an instant answer to the age-old question, "What should an average transcriptionist produce?" Next to "what's a line?" this question ranks at the top of identifying an individual as someone who is not a medical transcriptionist and is a prime candidate for Zig Ziglar-type salesmen who want to close a fast sale. The question is a dead giveaway.

AAMT's response to individuals who seek information regarding productivity standards is this: Accurate productivity standards should be developed from within an existing environment and should be based on the accumulated history of that environment (office, department, etc). We make suggestions on how to compile the necessary information that will enable them to develop their own productivity standards. The entrepreneurs who sell standards have come up with what the average transcriptionist should be able to accomplish under normal working conditions. In my 23 years of transcribing I have yet to meet anyone working in normal conditions or whom I consider to be an average MT because these terms are as ambiguous as a description of an average line.

Because supervisors and managers seek instant answers to their questions about productivity, they are easily sold on averages and normals. How easy it is to take the numbers provided and impose them on medical transcriptionists. Like small clothing stretched on a large frame, one size fits all can only be stretched to its limit before the seams split or the transcriptionists quit, and the supervisor/manager is left wondering what went wrong.

I've heard this kind of marketing and sales referred to as "transcription by the pound," an appropriate term indeed. If supervisors/managers are willing to subscribe to an average number of times the average transcriptionist with an average level of experience working in an average facility in an average city that is equipped with average medical technology should be able to pound in an average transcription hour, dictated by an average dictator with average dictation equipment, then I think we should explore a new incentive program and salary structure ... one that sells medical transcription by the pound. For instance, "I'll buy 6,000 pounds of average quality transcription done in average time for $.05 per pound." It could work its way into the farm-to-market price index. It could be a real deal ... cheaper than peanuts by the pound. My imagination can even envision a sale around the holidays or special markdowns for smooth-speaking dictators from 7 o'clock to 3 o'clock, Monday through Wednesday. There are all kinds of creative marketing ideas we could employ.

As long as the free enterprise system provides an opportunity to sell, there will be salesmen, and I support and defend their rights in that free system. A successful salesman can and will get a commission from almost any industry that has a need. Among the many needs of the medical transcription industry is a need for productivity standards. Anyone who has a knack for selling standards will profit from this need. As with any sale, the buyer needs to be alert to bottom lines and to the space in between the lines. Some of the questions I would pose to the sales representative of a line of average productivity standards are:

• Is the average medical transcriptionist educated, trained, or educated and trained? If so, for what length of time?

• Does the average medical transcriptionist have continuing education? If so, how much?

• Is the average medical transcriptionist certified? If not, does it matter?

• How much experience does the average medical transcriptionist have? If so, what kind of experience?

• Does the average medical transcriptionist do surgical reports? If so, how complicated are they?

• Does the average transcriptionist work in a two-person office or a 900-bed facility?

• Is the average medical transcriptionist responsible for correcting dictation errors?

- Does the average medical transcriptionist wear any other hats besides that of medical transcriptionist? If so, how is lost time evaluated and by whom?

- Is the average dictator English speaking or is English the dictator's second language?

- Does the average transcriptionist have quality standards? If so, are they industry standards or facility standards and are they consistent with each other?

- Who is the final authority on what is average anything?

And the list goes on.

The bottom line is that there is no such thing as a national average productivity standard, an average working environment, or an average transcriptionist. It is safe to say that there probably will never be.

It is unfortunate that a one-size-fits-all solution to this dilemma cannot be applied to medical transcriptionists. Hearing others defend the average, I am reminded of a physician-speaker who was asked to explain standard quality patient care. He drew in his breath and thoughtfully answered: "Well, you see, there is no such thing. There are variables that must be taken into consideration…" It's comforting to know that medical transcription is not alone in addressing standards issues and not the only profession which others would be comfortable in lumping into the number crunchers' game of averages.

Reprinted from JAAMT, *Vol. 11, No. 3, May-June 1992, pp. 12–13. Copyright 1992, AAMT, Modesto, CA.*

AAMT Position Paper:
Quality Assurance Guidelines

Issue

Establishing effective quality assurance guidelines in medical transcription. This position statement outlines key elements of an effective quality assurance program.

Issue summary

The patient's healthcare record assists physicians, insurance companies, researchers, future healthcare providers, and others in a variety of patient-related activities. Communicating correct patient information in a clear, consistent manner is essential, but adequate procedures to assure quality in medical transcription are lacking in some transcription environments because of perceived difficulties in measuring quality and the opinion that attention to quality will reduce productivity.

Policies and procedures generally exist for measuring *quantity,* and therefore, the income of many medical transcriptionists is dependent on the amount of transcription they produce. However, *quality* has a greater impact than quantity on effective communication. Establishing and measuring quality standards is a holistic process measured by the overall effectiveness of the document—unlike quantity, which can be measured only in numbers.

AAMT developed the following guidelines to provide the basis for quality assurance policies and to establish the importance of quality in patient care documentation. These guidelines are based on the premise that managers and supervisors dedicated to quality assurance must have an equal dedication to providing a quality work environment.

AAMT position

The demand to produce quality work requires adequate support. Up-to-date reference materials, adequate equipment, adequate dictating methods and equipment, continuing education, an ergonomically and psychologically safe work environment, and supervision by qualified medical transcriptionists are essential conditions for successful quality assurance in medical transcription. Transcriptionists cannot reasonably be expected to fulfill these quality guidelines if they are not provided with the necessary environment and resources to support quality assurance.

Quality Assurance for Medical Transcription

- Appropriate work environment and adequate resources are provided and maintained.

- Medical transcription services within (or for) the healthcare organization are performed and supervised by qualified medical transcriptionists.

- Designated equipment is utilized skillfully and efficiently, with proper guidelines and demonstration for use available to dictators and transcriptionists.

- Patient demographics are verified.

- Dictator identification is verified.

- Appropriate format is followed.

- English language rules are adopted and used consistently.

- Current reference materials are used consistently.

- Visual proofreading as well as electronic spell- and grammar-checking (if available) are performed.

- Obvious inconsistencies, discrepancies, and inaccuracies are recognized and appropriately revised, edited, or clarified, without altering the meaning of dictation or changing the dictator's style; flagged for dictator review; or brought to the attention of appropriate personnel for action.

- Appropriate personnel are consulted regarding dictation that may be considered unprofessional, frivolous, insulting, inflammatory, or inappropriate.

- Appropriate risk management personnel are consulted regarding unusual circumstances and/or information with possible risk factors.

- Reasonable deadlines are met.

- Appropriate measures are taken to protect patient confidentiality and system security.

- Administrative procedures are followed (e.g., copy distribution).

- If amendment or revision of the record is required, appropriate corrections or revisions are made according to established medicolegal guidelines, policies, and procedures.

- Document storage and retrieval guidelines are followed.

- A mechanism for feedback to the medical transcriptionist is provided.

- Random quality control review is performed by a qualified medical transcriptionist.

Position summary

A concern for quality need not override the goal of productivity. Inherent in these guidelines are provisions that assure not only prompt turnaround for transcription but also security, accuracy, and other quality concerns. However, these guidelines also assume that commitment to quality includes the willingness of employers to invest in the necessary resources. The qualified medical transcriptionist, given the proper environment and resources, will effectively balance quantity and quality concerns in order to produce in a reasonable amount of time a highly effective communication tool: the patient care document.

Adopted by AAMT House of Delegates, August 3, 1994.
Copyright 1994, AAMT, Modesto, CA.

Quality Assurance: Key to Cost Containment in Medical Transcription

Stella Olson, CMT

E veryone in the medical field knows that cost containment is a priority. How can medical transcriptionists contribute to cost containment? Is simply producing the most error-free medical report enough? Or do we also have the same responsibility as others in the allied health professions to assume a role in quality assurance?

We can contribute to cost containment of the finished medical report by building a sound quality assurance program into our transcription environments. Yes, quality assurance costs money, but in the overall picture it is essential to cost containment. A medical report with content errors, typos, grammar and punctuation errors, will at some time be returned for correction. The re-doing of that report will at least duplicate its original production cost—and in some instances it will escalate to two or three times that original cost. No physician in today's medical world wants his or her signature attached to an inadequate, error-ridden report. It is a reflection on the physician, the institution, the transcription department or service and, bottom line, the medical transcriptionist.

Medical transcriptionists are responsible for proofing their transcribed reports; however, the human element of error is always present. A second look at the transcribed report is a must. We can no longer contribute to "transcription by the pound." The transcribed medical report communicates information about a human being, and that person deserves the best that we can prepare.

Standards for quality assurance should be established. A quality assurance transcriptionist (QAT) with the status of certified medical transcriptionist, excellent listening skills, knowledge of grammar and punctuation, and the ability to give constructive feedback to every transcriptionist will not only place your transcription environment at its highest quality level but will bring to medical transcriptionists the acknowledgment as professionals that we want to attain.

Medical transcription practitioners have an obligation to provide quality assurance. It may not be possible to listen to every dictated word, but there are ways and means by which quality assurance on a continued basis can be established.

For new employees or entry-level medical transcriptionists, it is necessary to listen to the dictation as their work is reviewed. No history of quality levels for these individuals exists. Every transcriptionist has a different pace, but at the end of a 90-day period the QAT will have a clear picture of the current and potential quality of an individual's transcription.

Once the medical transcriptionist has established credibility in quality production, proofing on the CRT screen instead of the printed report is the most cost-effective way to assure quality. Paper waste, printer ribbon waste, and unnecessary reprints are eliminated, and listening time is reduced. The QAT listens only for flagged blanks, garbled dictation, or for clarification.

The QAT then provides constructive suggestions to the transcriptionists for improving their quality control, as well as for continuing education purposes.

Internal audits of all medical transcriptionists are the final step in providing quality assurance with a goal of an 80 to 100 accuracy score. The internal audit becomes part of the medical transcriptionist's evaluation process. This procedure also adds to the credibility of your transcription department or service and to your well-earned status as professionals.

Individual internal audits are as confidential as personnel records and medical reports. Collectively, they are a measure by which the quality of a transcription department or service is gauged. They also contribute to the development of a cost-contained department or service.

Following are examples of a proofreading statement and an audit statement and log, along with scores for internal audit.

PROOFREADING STATEMENT

MT/CMT name: _____

Client: _____

Date proofed: _____

Date transcribed: _____

Total pages/document name: _____

Findings: _____

_____

_____

_____

Proofreader: _____

MT/CMT signature: _____

AUDIT STATEMENT

MT's name: _____

Date of audit: _____

Account: _____

Document name: _____

Character count: _____

Line count w/o blanks: _____

Total pages: _____

Total number of errors: _____

Additional comments: _____

_____

Employee's signature: _____

Date: _____

AUDIT LOG SHEET

Date	MT's Initials	Document Name	Auditor's Initials

SCORING SYSTEM FOR INTERNAL AUDIT

Major errors:	content only	1 point
Minor errors:	punctuation, paragraph assembly, grammar	½ point
	transposed letters, letters left out of words	¼ point

	score
0 points per 100 lines without blank lines	100
1 point per 100 lines without blank lines	90
2 points per 100 lines without blank lines	80
3 points per 100 lines without blank lines	70
4 points per 100 lines without blank lines	60

Any audit with a score of 70 or below:
MT needs to study more and must be audited
again within 30 days to evaluate.

All audit sheets are submitted to the manager or department head on completion for review. Employees who are audited can then be interviewed and the results of the audit discussed. Audit sheets then become part of the medical transcriptionist's personnel records, and a schedule is developed by personnel for the next audit. A complete audit schedule is given to the audit supervisor for future reference.

Reprinted from JAAMT, *Vol. 11, No. 3, May-June 1992, pp. 32-33. Copyright 1992, Modesto, CA.*

Appendix W

The Quality of Patient Care Documentation

Claudia Tessier, CAE, CMT, RRA

Author's note: The following is adapted from communications that AAMT directed to participants in a series of meetings initiated by the American Health Information Management Association (AHIMA) and including representatives from a variety of healthcare associations and environments; copies were also sent to the Joint Commission on Accreditation of Healthcare Organizations (JCAHO) and to the Healthcare Financing Administration (HCFA) of the U.S. Department of Health and Human Services.

AAMT is concerned that discussions to date related to authentication, signatures, and authorship have emphasized the reduction of administrative burdens (incomplete records; JCAHO type I contingencies; HCFA citations). We urge that all involved take care that this focus does not distract us from the essential issue: the quality of healthcare communications, i.e., patient care documentation and, thus, patient care (as well as reimbursement, research, statistics, and legal pursuits, of course) which is based on and related to that documentation. With this document and accompanying materials, we will attempt to demonstrate the degree to which the quality of patient care documentation is influenced by the processes related to its preparation and why those processes must be addressed and improved if patient care documentation is to improve and if protection of patients' rights is to be assured.

Authorship, as defined by AHIMA, is the "process whereby the healthcare provider reviews documentation, prior to release for patient care, to assure quality and accuracy." With or without signature (electronic or traditional), this is not presently achievable, and to achieve it will require dramatic changes in how healthcare providers input their reports, how those reports are prepared for output, and when those reports are reviewed by the healthcare provider.

We believe that to achieve the highest quality of patient care documentation will require real-time documentation, which we define as input (dictation) at the point of care, concurrent transcription (by voice recognition with the assistance of a medical transcriptionist or directly by a medical transcriptionist), review and editing by the transcriptionist to achieve essential characteristics, immediate transmittal to the originator for review (and correction if necessary), and finally authentication. Although we are far from achieving real-time documentation, the healthcare community is in a good position to develop it in its best potential form if we take a realistic view of current documentation practices and processes, determine the necessary changes to achieve our goals, and prepare a realistic plan for implementing those changes.

In this regard, we are prepared to work closely with associations representing physicians and other healthcare providers who dictate, in order to effect real-time documentation as described above. We must break down the barriers between medical transcriptionists and dictators so that they can work together cooperatively and freely to assure that patient documentation as prepared through the dictation/ transcription process is of the highest quality at the time it is incorporated into the patient record—much as laboratory technicians work with pathologists and labora- tory directors to assure that laboratory reports are accurate at the time they are reported and sent to the record.

The expertise of medical transcriptionists (MTs) is unmatched when it comes to the dictation/transcription process for patient care documentation. We recognize that others are experts about other documentation processes, e.g., phone orders for drugs. We urge that all related and interested parties be included in the exploration of these issues sooner rather than later. Their involvement will not only encourage the ultimate acceptance of proposed changes and solutions but will enhance its ultimate value as well. Further, we urge the involvement of patient representatives in order to assure that patients are informed and that their interests, concerns, and rights are addressed.

Note: As we address "authorship," the issue of electronic signatures and their misuse remains unfinished. AAMT wants the record to show that (1) we support the use of an electronic signature by the person whose signature it represents, and (2) we oppose the delegation of the responsibility and authority to drop in an electronic signature (or use a rubber stamp) to a medical transcriptionist or anyone else. The use of electronic signatures continues to be delegated, and so the issue remains one of concern not only to medical transcriptionists but to the fundamental issue of the quality of patient care documentation.

Characteristics of quality patient care documentation

AAMT summarizes the characteristics (the 7 C's) of patient care documentation, particularly as they apply to dictation and transcription, as follows, acknowledging that their applicability and use may vary in differing contexts.

complete

All required, desired, and relevant information is presented. This includes essen- tial components of the patient record as a whole, as well as each of its documents. In the transition to electronic recordkeeping, it is anticipated that information will not be repeated in multiple reports if it can be readily and meaningfully retrieved upon command from other parts of the record.

consistent

All information is consistent internally within the specific report and externally with the remainder of the patient record. Contradictory information must be flagged and resolved in a manner and format that provides for audit trails and assures that accurate information is readily identifiable and retrievable and that inaccurate information is clearly labeled as such.

clear

The information is readable and readily understandable for use by concurrent and future healthcare providers, for reimbursement, for statistical and research uses, and for legal purposes. The assurance of clarity requires attention to structure, format, organization, grammar, syntax, language usage, as well as avoidance of redundancy.

correct

The report is accurate in content and presentation. This includes patient and provider identification accuracy and content accuracy, as well as spelling, grammar, syntax, and organizational accuracy.

confidential

The patient's rights to confidentiality and privacy are protected throughout the preparation (dictation and transcription), storage, maintenance, and usage of the documentation. Security of the documentation must be defined and refined, including but not limited to authorized access. Those who delegate authorized access must be held accountable.

concurrent

The documentation is dictated, transcribed, authenticated, and incorporated into the patient record in a timely manner. The goal is to achieve as close to real-time documentation as possible without jeopardizing any of the other characteristics.

credible

The system provides realistic means for achieving quality documentation, including the inevitable need for corrections. A mechanism for "lockout" is needed to prevent unauthorized access and changes and to provide an audit trail of authorized access and changes.

Appropriate attention to these characteristics for documentation provides a strong basis for determining the most appropriate future care. It also assists in risk management, reducing the legal liability of all concerned. Additionally, it promotes appropriate and timely reimbursement, provides accurate statistics and research data, and fulfills the role of the patient record as a legal document.

Unfortunately, these characteristics of patient care documentation do not always reflect reality in relation to dictation and transcription. The reasons they may fall short are myriad and far-reaching. To appreciate this, one must understand the processes of dictation and transcription and the related problems that may arise. Some of these are discussed below. (Note: Not all of these characteristics apply to all dictation or all transcription at all times.)

Examples of dictation problems

Dictation is a skill that does not come readily to most people. Few healthcare providers are taught how to dictate, and few take to it naturally. So, dictation tends to be done as spontaneous, stream-of-consciousness speech rather than as prepared, organized, and clear speech. For English-as-a-second-language providers, there is the added challenge of communicating in a non-native language.

Much dictation does not include certain required information, and the information that is provided is oftentimes inaccurate, inadequate, unclear, inconsistent.

Dictation is frequently done with background noise such as family arguments, phones ringing, dogs barking, freeway traffic. The dictator is often doing other things, such as eating, listening to music, driving a car, even going to the bathroom. Any sounds other than the dictation itself obscure dictation. Dictation may be mumbled, muffled, excessively soft or loud, slow or fast. The tone and pitch of the dictating voice also influence the degree to which it can be understood.

Much dictation equipment is inadequate or outdated, or it is not used properly, thus diminishing rather than enhancing sound quality or cutting off dictation.

Much dictation is done without access to the patient's record, a practice that diminishes accuracy, consistency, and clarity.

Dictation frequently includes new, slang, personally coined, or difficult-to-document terminology. Soundalikes are a particular challenge, for example *cabbage* becomes *CABG*. The expanse of medical language is growing, and dictation tends to attract new terminology. Few terms are spelled, and often those words that are, are spelled incorrectly. Additionally, the use of abbreviations in dictation is rampant, and a single abbreviation may have multiple meanings, further obscuring communication.

Even when patients are correctly identified, their names may not be spelled correctly (or at all). Other demographic information may not be accurate. Occasionally, dictation is done on the wrong patient.

Most dictators take appropriate precautions to protect patient confidentiality, but some dictation is done where it can be overheard by those who should not be privy to confidential patient information. Though not done deliberately, the negative effects are not dependent on intent. Also of increasing concern is the use of cellular phones as dictation instruments; these provide no security whatsoever.

Some dictation is done days, weeks, even months after the event. Some dictators instruct transcriptionists to date reports when they should have been dictated rather than when they were actually done. Some histories and physicals are dictated a month or more prior to surgery, leading to outdated and often misplaced documentation.

Sometimes reports are dictated by other than the responsible caregiver, and the dictator "pretends" to be that caregiver. The MT who recognizes this subterfuge is expected in some instances to ignore it.

Many transcribed reports are signed/authenticated long after they have been prepared and oftentimes without being reviewed for accuracy. Blanks and inconsistencies often remain.

Examples of transcription problems

Transcription is the process of translating the spoken word to the printed word (paper-based or computer-based). Because most people speak differently than they write and read, dictation cannot be transcribed verbatim. It must be translated from the spoken word to written form; this requires interpretation and editing. (See chart at end for some examples that contrast verbatim dictation with edited transcription.)

Qualified MTs recognize internal inconsistencies, and if they transcribed earlier reports for a particular patient, they may recognize inconsistencies with those as well. They decipher dictation that is not clear (due to sound or dictation quality), edit for grammar and syntax, reorganize content, research new or unfamiliar terminology, make obvious corrections, and translate abbreviations when their meanings can be determined. As they edit, they take care not to change the meaning of the dictation or the style of the dictators. They leave blanks when unclear or inconsistent dictation cannot be resolved and when they are not confident that what they hear is what was intended.

Some dictation is so poor that it cannot be deciphered. Some background noise is so loud, the dictation cannot be separated from it.

Many work environments provide inadequate and outdated references, making it difficult for MTs to research new, unfamiliar, or difficult-to-find terminology.

Most MTs are discouraged (sometimes restricted) from making direct contact with dictators, who could be their best resource for clarification and for assuring the highest quality of documentation.

When English is a second language for those who are dictating, MTs must not only interpret the effect of their accents but sometimes their sentence structure as well, which may be based on that of their native language. Some MTs become especially adept with certain accents. Regional accents among U.S.-born natives may also present a challenge.

Many MTs are supervised by non-MTs who make demands for quantity at the expense of quality. This is due partly to their not understanding the characteristics, the process, or the requirements related to dictation and transcription, and partly to quantitative demands made on them in turn.

Outdated or inadequate transcription and word processing equipment inhibits the sound quality of dictation and obstructs the timely preparation of transcripts.

Some institutions select MTs on the basis of their keyboard skills rather than their medical and English language skills and their editorial ability. These employers may want verbatim transcription, which guarantees the diminished quality of patient care documentation. Further, unqualified MTs leave blanks that qualified MTs would know how to fill. (AAMT's *Model Job Description* illustrates the complex qualifications for doing medical transcription.)

Many MTs are paid by the amount of transcription they do, as measured by whatever base unit the employer or supervisor sets, e.g., bits, bytes, characters, words, lines, reports, minutes of dictation. They are penalized for taking time to prepare reports with the characteristics necessary to assure quality. Some MTs are directed to transcribe verbatim, to make their best guess, to leave no blanks, to ignore inconsistencies, and to meet quotas.

Although MTs regularly seek feedback about unclear or inconsistent dictation, and about new terminology (to complete the report in question, to further their professional development, and to assist in preparing future transcripts by the same physician), they seldom get such feedback. Some flags prepared by the MTs may have dropped off or been removed by the time the report reaches the originator; others are ignored. (*Note:* Because feedback to MTs about reports they have flagged is so skimpy, AAMT is particularly concerned by proposals to assume authentication has occurred unless the author notes discrepancies or provides corrections within seven days of receiving the report. We are also concerned about how subsequent caregivers will be able to distinguish between an original report and a corrected report. When we posed this concern to a major medical center using this type of system, they admitted the system was faulty: they could easily mark the corrected report as such, but they could not always assure that the inaccurate original report and all its copies were marked in a way that would assure it would not be assumed to be the only such report.)

Most MTs take care to protect patient confidentiality, but this is not always in their control. Telecommunicating, for example, increases the risk for breaches of confidentiality; a report prepared at a contract service may be printed at a healthcare site, where it may be viewed (and even changed, as some are) by clerks and others, oftentimes without the knowledge of the contract service or medical transcriptionist who prepared the report.

Some supervisors and employers direct medical transcriptionists to change the date of dictation and/or transcription so that it appears the work was done when it was supposed to have been done although the actual date(s) may be days, weeks, or months later.

Some MTs report that they continue to be told to drop in electronic signatures, even when the institution's printed policies restrict this.

And the list goes on.

Summary

Medical transcriptionists can attest to the accuracy of their transcription, but they cannot attest to the accuracy of patient or provider identification. The quality of patient care documentation can only be attested to by provider review and signature, i.e., through authentication.

Sample Medical Dictation

Sample actual physician dictation transcribed verbatim (a.k.a. voice recognition)	Edited transcription
The patient is to remain plastered for the next six to eight weeks.	The patient is to remain in a plaster cast for the next six to eight weeks.
I scrounged around in the blood vessel.	I explored the blood vessel.
She was confused on admission, but over the past five days her mental status has cleared and now she's complaining about everything.	She was confused on admission, but over the past five days her mental status has cleared. She now has several complaints.
The patient was treated with enemas and laxatives by mouth.	The patient was treated with enemas and oral laxatives.
The tourniquet was placed and the leg inflated.	The tourniquet was placed on the leg and inflated.
She was treated with Mycostatin oral suppositories.	She was treated with Mycostatin oral suspension.
The culture grew out Staph epididymis.	The culture grew out Staphylococcus epidermidis.
The patient was treated with nitroglycerin and sublingual lidocaine.	The patient was treated with lidocaine and sublingual nitroglycerin.
The patient has bilateral swelling in both lower ankles.	The patient has bilateral ankle swelling.
Urinary system: Denies dyspnea.	Urinary system: Denies dysuria.

Bilaterally descended phallus.

Bilaterally descended testicles.

Teeth are edentulous.

Mouth is edentulous.

Clear to auscultation, without rales, rhonchi, or breathing.

Clear to auscultation, without rales, rhonchi, or wheezes.

The patient's left leg felt less sensible.

There was decreased sensation in the patient's left leg.

The patient had bilateral hysterectomy and oophorectomy.

The patient had hysterectomy and bilateral oophorectomy.

The patient had chest pain every day for one to two times per day for the last four to five days.

The patient has had daily chest pain for the last four to five days, occurring one to two times per day.

He had a left toe amputation one month ago; he also had a left above-the-knee amputation last year.

(Transcriptionist must check with physician or review chart further, since dictation indicates an impossible situation.)

By physicians who speak English as a second language:

She goes twice weekly for traction and to get her legs pulled.

She goes twice weekly for leg traction.

The patient has a rectal disorderment.

The patient has a rectal disorder.

There is no headal or truncal tremor.

There is no cephalic or truncal tremor.
or
There is no tremor of the head or trunk.

The patient is discomfortable.

The patient is uncomfortable.

Total Quality Management and Medical Transcription

Claudia Tessier, CAE, CMT, RRA

The Joint Commission on Accreditation of Healthcare Organizations (JCAHO) is requiring hospitals to participate in continuous quality improvement (CQI) by 1994. CQI is the healthcare version of total quality management (TQM), a universal management system based on the concept that ongoing improvement involves everybody. It takes a process-oriented approach rather than a results-oriented one, and its adoption by the healthcare industry provides a unique opportunity for medical transcriptionists' long-standing commitment to quality to be valued.

W. Edwards Deming, generally considered the father of TQM, has identified 14 TQM points that are essential for implementing the system. Following is an introduction to TQM's 14 points as they apply to medical transcription:

1. Establish constancy of purpose.

Everyone involved in the TQM organization cooperates in the efforts toward achieving quality. Thus, when a healthcare institution or medical transcription service adopts TQM, medical transcription will be included.

2. Adopt the new philosophy.

Adopting the TQM philosophy means shifting the paradigm for medical transcription from "how much" to "how well." According to Deming, 85% of the problems in an organization are caused by the system's management, not by the system's employees. With TQM, MTs need no longer bear the sole burden for "too little, too late, too wrong" transcription. Rather, they will have the opportunity and responsibility to work with management to identify problems and solutions.

3. Stop depending on mass inspection; improve processes instead.

TQM rejects incentive programs that utilize inspection as a means to penalize the employee, even to reduce wages; programs that emphasize what is wrong and who made it wrong instead of why it is wrong and what can be changed to avoid the same mistake in the future. With TQM, management and MTs will work together to improve the process so as to improve the quality, not to make MTs hit the keyboard faster.

4. Stop awarding business on the basis of price alone.

Decision-makers in TQM systems recognize the value of what their dollar is going to buy, whether it is a dollar spent on an MT employee or a dollar spent on a medical transcription service. Deming advocates achievement of quality through long-term relationships with suppliers. The parties work together to improve the process so as to enhance the quality, and everyone wins.

5. Improve constantly and forever every system of production and service.

TQM advocates don't wait for it to be "broke" to fix it. They constantly seek ways to reduce waste and improve the quality of medical transcription by improving the process. Is equipment adequate and well maintained? Are medical references current? Are sufficient references available? Are new and difficult-to-find terminology lists developed and shared? Etc., etc., etc. TQM recognizes that it costs less to improve the process than to redo work that doesn't meet standards.

6. Use modern methods of training.

TQM advocates the development of comprehensive and integrated staff training programs. Total quality managers will assist MT students, entry-level MTs, and long-term MTs to improve in order to work toward closing the gap between MT supply and demand.

7. Institute leadership.

TQM recognizes that leadership is developed at all levels, not just the top, and it seeks to eliminate the bean counter mentality. For medical transcription, this means supervisors will be more than line (or character or byte, etc.) counters. They will work with MTs to improve the system so MTs can do their jobs to the best of their ability and develop the ability to do it better. They will encourage MTs to take leadership roles in identifying ways to improve the process in order to improve quality.

8. Drive out fears.

TQM managers drive out the fears of employees. A major fear of MTs working in incentive programs that place quantity before quality is not having enough hours and enough endurance to produce enough lines (or other units of measure) to meet productivity demands that will pay them enough to meet their needs. TQM will help MTs feel secure in order to be motivated to improve the quality and productivity of transcription.

9. Break down barriers between departments and staff areas.

Under TQM, medical transcriptionists will be encouraged to interact with other individuals and departments that need their services and can assist them in fulfilling their responsibilities. Because TQM values cooperation, it will promote MTs working *with* rather than *for* other healthcare professionals and encourage MTs helping one another without fear of losing pay due to decreased productivity.

10. Eliminate slogans, exhortations, and targets for the workforce.

TQM avoids slogans, exhortations, and targets because they too often represent an effort on management's part to put the blame on individual employees rather than on the system. TQM requires the commitment of management and their cooperation with employees, including MTs.

11. Eliminate numerical quotas. Substitute leadership.

The value of healthcare is not measured by the numbers and neither should quality medical transcription. Quantity goals, which inherently focus on the end result, will be replaced by quality goals, which focus on the process. This supports AAMT's long-standing conviction that there is no average line count for MTs and there is no national productivity standard for MTs. TQM recognizes the impact of variables on productivity and seeks to minimize these variables as a means to improve the process and therefore the quality (and quantity).

12. Remove obstacles to employees' pride of workmanship.

TQM seeks to identify and remove obstacles: inadequate equipment and resources, outdated reference materials, and outdated policies and procedures that restrict MTs from doing their best. Other obstacles include inappropriate job classifications, titles, descriptions, and salaries.

13. Begin a vigorous program of education and self-improvement.

TQM will provide MTs with opportunities for increasing their knowledge, their leadership abilities, and their individual talents. In a TQM system, MTs will be encouraged to become involved in their professional association, to attend and participate in conferences and educational programs, and to earn the credential of certified medical transcriptionist. And these accomplishments will be recognized by the employer.

14. Put everybody in the organization to work to accomplish the transformation to quality.

Total quality management creates and maintains an environment that promotes cooperation among all employees, including MTs, toward constantly seeking to improve quality.

Deming tells us that when quality comes first, productivity follows. AAMT has consistently promoted this concept. MTs are proud of what they do. A document full of inaccuracies is likely to be the only reflection of the quality of healthcare a patient has received, and more important, will contribute to decision-making related to the care that patient will receive. In addition, it may determine the outcome of a legal battle. Certainly, it is of considerable importance that it represents the institution responsible for the care of the patient.

TQM will provide MTs an opportunity to improve the quality of healthcare through quality communication of quality information.

Reprinted from JAAMT, Vol. 11, No. 5, September-October 1992, pp. 4–5. Copyright 1992, AAMT, Modesto, CA.

Appendix Y

Medical Language

John H. Dirckx, MD

Q   In your column and elsewhere I often see medical terms called "irregular" or "incorrect," including ones that are in constant use and are in all the dictionaries. Who ultimately decides whether a medical term is right or wrong? Are there official committees that rule on these things? Can a correct term become wrong or vice versa?

A   A term or expression can be judged right or wrong, apt or unacceptable, regular or deviant according to a variety of standards, the most important of which are listed below.

    1. In applying the standard of usage, one inquires how widely a language practice is accepted by the community of language users. This is the standard that most modern dictionaries, including medical dictionaries, seek to establish. It is important to recognize, however, that the most diligent lexicographer cannot claim to have sampled more than an infinitesimal fraction of the actual language practices of a population, and that by the time a dictionary has been printed and distributed, its assessments of usage may already be somewhat out of date. Despite these short-comings, dictionaries and other reference works (glossaries, grammars, style manuals) that purport to record current usage are the most useful and reliable authorities available to writers, editors, and medical transcriptionists.

    2. One can also apply an *etymologic* or historical standard, asking how faithfully a word preserves the form and meaning of its earliest known origins. By this standard, a great many of our most-used technical terms, including all of those based on metaphor (**cervix** 'neck', cardiac **chamber**, **muscle** 'little mouse') could be judged aberrant. Persons who assign primary importance to etymologic standards of correctness overlook the fact that daily usage is constantly revising the pronunciation, spelling, and connotations of many words and so moving them ever further from their historical roots and traditional associations. Even if it were desirable to prevent this morphologic and semantic drift, it would scarcely be possible. In addition, no linguist can trace the history of any word further back than the earliest written records—about 6,000 years—whereas human beings have probably been talking for at least ten times that long. In contrast to the usual lexicographic practice of former generations, modern dictionaries give little weight to etymologic considerations in recording the forms and meanings of words. Incidentally, the growth of scientific knowledge sometimes reveals that the etymologic sense of a term is not as apt or true as was once believed. For example, **atom,** a term borrowed from ancient Greek science and meaning 'indivisible particle', has been shown by the splitting of the atom to be a misnomer.

3. There is also a standard of *consistency* or analogy, based on the extent to which a language practice complies with general patterns of spelling, pronunciation, word formation, or meaning. Practices that do not fit the expected pattern may be designated "irregular," but that does not prevent many of them from remaining in constant use, particularly when more regular forms are not available. Morphologically irregular terms such as **distention, funduscopic, heparin, iritis, luetic, metastasize, myositis, presbycusis, sinusitis,** and **tyrosine** have become so firmly established that only a crank would object to their continued use. Sometimes a word that appears to deviate from the pattern of similar words is found to be in perfect accord with some other pattern or model, which has governed its formation.

4. A *pragmatic* or utilitarian standard considers how efficiently and unequivocally a word or usage serves its primary function as a medium of communication. In this perspective, vague or ambiguous expressions such as **factor, normal, small bowel cancer**, and "Warts on the other hand are contagious" might be found less suitable than more specific and unequivocal ones such as **cause, unimpaired, small-bowel cancer**, and "Warts, on the other hand, are contagious."

5. Some like to apply a criterion they call *logic* to language practices. By this yardstick, for example, **first two** is logical but **two first** is not; **the twin born later** is logical but **the twin born last** is not; **a reason for his remaining dyspneic** is logical but **for him remaining dyspneic** is not; and so forth. Although many such arguments make sense to a majority of observers, some of them seem to suggest that one person's logic is another person's nonsense. Language practices evolve in response to the need of speakers and writers to make themselves understood. Where this development diverges uniformly from what seems to be a strict logical path, it is probably the logic that should be called in question.

6. A word or usage can be judged, or rather ranked, with respect to the level of *formality* in speech and writing to which it most fittingly corresponds. While many expressions are at home in any level, some (**endeavor, presuppose, sustain, tranquil**) usually appear only in fairly formal settings, and others (**bust, dickens, not about to, plan on going**) are appropriate only in more colloquial contexts. The transcriptionist must often apply this standard in judging whether dictated material should be transcribed verbatim or rendered in more formal language.

7. Related to the foregoing is the standard of *propriety* or decency, according to which certain words or phrases are tabooed as vulgar, profane, obscene, or offensive to certain groups or class of persons.

8. An *esthetic* standard takes into account such abstract qualities of language as poetic imagery, rhythm, and euphony. The application of such standards is highly subjective at best and often becomes a matter of individual taste. Grammarians of the old school based many of their rules, some of which survive today, on such considerations. For example, some still favor the rule that forbids adding the comparative suffix *-er* or the superlative *-est* to adjectives of more than one syllable. According to this rule, **most common** is preferable to **commonest**.

9. There is also a *social* standard, according to which the language practices of educated and cultivated persons are automatically assumed to be correct, and deviations from these practices are condemned as "substandard." But who is entitled to decide for the rest of us what is "refined" or "educated" language? Lexicographers used to assume this authority, but few modern dictionaries contain usage labels based strictly on upper-class speech and writing practices.

10. The nomenclatures of certain basic sciences and branches of medicine have been defined within fairly narrow limits by various official or quasi-official boards and associations. The spelling and meaning of terms pertaining to anatomy, histology, embryology, chemistry, pharmacology (both generic names and brand names), and the taxonomy of plants (including pathogenic bacteria and fungi) and animals (including parasites and disease vectors) have been fixed in this way. Some medical specialty boards and government agencies have established official definitions for terms concerning their areas of interest or influence. For example, the *Diagnostic and Statistical Manual of Mental Disorders* published by the American Psychiatric Association contains definitions, in the form of diagnostic criteria, for all currently recognized mental diseases. Although these official nomenclatures are widely accepted and are recorded in technical dictionaries and other reference works, changes in official terminology penetrate very slowly into workaday medical speech and writing. For example, eponymic terms such as **fallopian tube** and **eustachian tube**, which were rejected from anatomic terminology several decades ago, continue in wide use in preference to the official **uterine tube** and **auditory tube**.

11. Because there is a strong subjective element in our experience and perception of language, few of us can resist using our own language practices as the ultimate test of correctness.

Although each of the criteria of aptness or correctness listed above has its own kind of validity, none of them can be applied in an arbitrary or absolute way, much less enforced. Some of these standards overlap others, while, on the other hand, some criteria of correctness are incompatible with other criteria. In judging whether a given language practice is right or wrong, one should evaluate it in the light of relevant circumstances, consult appropriate reference works, decide which standards are applicable, and try to assign each its due weight.

Reprinted from "Medical Language," JAAMT, Vol. 11, No. 3, May-June 1992, pp. 16–17. Copyright 1992, AAMT, Modesto, CA.

Debunking False Assumptions about Quality Management

Claudia Tessier, CAE, CMT, RRA

A AMT's continuing attention to quality reflects both our fundamental commitment to the value of accurate patient-care documentation as well as our responsiveness to what MTs, both members and nonmembers, tell us about unreasonable and inappropriate demands placed on them for quantity before quality. We want to assist MTs in persuading their supervisors, managers, and employers that quality counts.

Where resistance to placing quality before quantity is met, it is likely due to the false assumptions about quality that Philip Crosby refutes in his popular management book *Quality is Free: The Art of Making Quality Certain* (Mentor Books, New American Library, New York, 1979).

Let's look at the erroneous assumptions about quality that Crosby describes and apply his arguments against them to the MT environment.

- **Erroneous assumption #1:** Quality means goodness, or luxury, or shininess, or weight.

Crosby points out that this assumption makes a cliché of quality. This allows both the MT and the supervisor/manager/employer to make personal assumptions about the definition of quality, thereby assuring inconsistency of goals and divergence of achievement. Debunking this assumption requires defining quality so that it can be managed. Crosby's definition of quality is "quality is conformance to requirements." By specifying those requirements for medical transcription, we can measure them in order to determine conformance. MT requirements for quality patient-care documentation include completeness, consistency, clarity, and correctness. These qualities recognize medical transcription as communication. (For a complete discussion of these qualities, see Appendix L, "Medical Transcription as Communication.") Of course, another measure of quality is productivity, but that measure must incorporate and cannot be isolated from communication qualities. Of what value is any amount of incomplete, inconsistent, unclear, or incorrect transcription whether produced quickly or slowly?

- **Erroneous assumption #2:** Quality is an intangible and therefore not measureable.

This false assumption allows MTs and MT supervisors/managers/employers to dismiss quality as something beyond their ability to measure. Crosby says the cost of quality is the expense of nonconformance—the cost of doing things wrong. For medical transcription, these costs include diminished and/or inappropriate patient care, inaccurate (and likely insufficient) reimbursement, increased liability for the healthcare institution as well as the healthcare providers, and inaccurate, incomplete statistics. Also included is the cost of redoing what could have been done right in the first place.

• **Erroneous assumption #3:** There is an "economics" of quality.

It is not unusual to hear MT supervisors/managers/employers describe medical transcription as "different" from other departments or businesses, meaning they cannot afford the cost or economics of quality. Crosby says this is typical. Each industry thinks it is different, but this means that they don't really understand quality. Countering this false assumption requires emphasizing again the meaning of quality (conformance to requirements) and pointing out that it is always cheaper to do some-thing right the first time. If MT supervisors/managers/employers want to be sure they are using the least expensive process then they need to understand the process itself, i.e., medical transcription, and how to measure it (see erroneous assumption #2). Understanding the process means understanding that medical transcription is not a keyboard skill but a language skill that uses technology as the vehicle for translating the language in its spoken form to printed form (whether "printed" on paper or on screen).

• **Erroneous assumption #4:** All the problems of quality are originated by the workers.

This assumption, of course, allows the blame for poor quality medical transcrip-tion to be placed squarely and totally on MTs. This avoidance technique permits supervisors/managers/employers to ignore their own deficiencies as well as those of their administrators, their accountants, their salespersons, their marketing personnel, etc., and to focus on the MTs themselves. Crosby reminds us that the workers (i.e., MTs) can contribute little to prevention of problems and to improved quality if all planning and decision making is done elsewhere. When MTs are involved with supervisors/managers/employers in planning, in setting policies, in making decisions, and in problem-solving, and when communication exists across traditional barriers, everyone is accountable for and committed to quality. The concept of blame is set aside and replaced by the concept of accountability for continuous quality improve-ment through cooperation of all parties.

- **Erroneous assumption #5:** Quality originates in the quality department.

This erroneous assumption is related to #4, but in this instance, the blame for inadequate quality is placed on (and accepted by) quality supervisors or quality assurance coordinators. They become burdened with the responsibility of identifying and correcting problems but are not given the authority to make changes toward improvement. Instead they continue to correct the same problems over and over because they don't have the influence to make lasting changes. MT quality reviewers must insist on having the authority to call problems by the names of those who create them, whether they be accountants, salespersons, supervisors, MTs, health information managers, owners, physicians, or others. They must have the confidence to report problems clearly and objectively, with recommendations for improvement, even when those recommendations will require fundamental shifts in policy and/or philosophy. Otherwise, they will continue to be held responsible for ensuring quality medical transcription without having the authority to resolve problems for which they themselves are not responsible.

Crosby tells us that quality management is "a management discipline concerned with preventing problems from occurring by creating the attitudes and controls that make prevention possible." Quality counts for medical transcription when all parties involved cooperate toward patient-care documentation that is complete, consistent, clear, and correct.

Reprinted from "Executive Message," JAAMT, Vol. 12, No. 1, January-February 1993, pp. 4–5. Copyright 1993, AAMT, Modesto, CA.

The Empowered Transcriptionist: A Valued Member of the Health Records Team

Claire R. Jacobsen, CMT

Misericordia Hospital is a 540-bed acute care teaching healthcare facility located in Edmonton, Alberta, Canada. Medical transcription is part of the health records department and has a staff of 6.9 FTE transcriptionists (11 full- and part-time staff) and 1 FTE clerk (2 part-time). Radiology and pathology have their own transcription services.

The health records team consists of a director, three area coordinators (health record services, medical transcription, and coding & data analysis), health record administrators, health record technicians, clerks, and a department secretary. All work together as a team to ensure that services provided are of the highest possible calibre. We are fortunate in that there is no sense of hierarchy.

Our teamwork extends beyond the workplace. We also play hard together and have won contests in the hospital such as Christmas decorating, pumpkin carving, and events in the team olympics held during Recognition Week. There is a lot of laughter in our department to go along with the ongoing hard work.

The medical transcriptionists have recently updated their job description to incorporate some of the excellent suggestions found in the AAMT model job description. They worked as a group, with input from all staff, and together developed and agreed to standards for transcription. They also helped develop standard formats to be used for various types of medical reports. The quality of work is exceptional, and standards are being met.

The transcriptionists continuously monitor their own quality and also practice partner proofreading which helps them identify areas for improvement. The partner system ensures that everyone has the same interpretation of formats, and it acts as a teaching tool.

Transcriptionists all help in the training of new staff and routinely help each other with difficult dictation. Group conferences happen spontaneously to help decipher dictation by some of our resident members. All staff are expected to maintain a notebook of new terminology and to share this with the other transcriptionists. This helps with our ongoing continuing education. We also arrange for physicians to come into the department once a month to talk about their speciality. Staff also have the opportunity to attend medical or surgical rounds.

The medical transcriptionists plan their own work day in accordance with department guidelines and assign their own work. They know what needs to be done first, and everyone is trained on all types of work. Consults, histories, operative notes, reports of delivery, and referral letters are priority items and are transcribed within

24 hours. All staff work on these reports first; then they move on to discharge summaries, which have a 72-hour turnaround time standard. This method seems to work very well as our priority work is always up to date. Consults often are on the patient chart within 10 minutes of the doctor having finished the dictation.

The staff enjoy having a variety of reports. Productivity is high as the transcriptionists are able to pace themselves and work on difficult dictation when they are at their peak level of performance, switching over to less demanding dictation when they feel the need for a break.

We feel that the people actually doing the work know best how to handle it. My position is not that of a supervisor but rather that of a coach and teacher. I am there as a resource person to provide answers to questions and give guidance when required. Employees are encouraged to make suggestions, and they have input into all decisions made. They have helped decide on the type of dictation system, office furniture, chairs, blinds, and reference materials that are used in the medical transcription area. They also have some input into the selection process for new transcriptionists.

Staff enjoy flex time as well. New daytime employees choose their starting time, any time from 0600 to 1000. The afternoon shift is allowed to start work early on Friday so that they can leave by 1930 that day.

We have monthly staff meetings in which staff are brought up to date on decisions and happenings throughout the hospital. The transcriptionists help prepare the agenda for the meeting, during which we discuss current issues and begin the problem-solving process. Each meeting includes a review of formats and procedures. We regularly provide a punctuation and grammar review and do some fun exercises as learning guides. We have two delightful references that we use (*The Transitive Vampire—a handbook of grammar for the Innocent, the Eager, and the Doomed*, and *The Well-Tempered Sentence—a punctuation handbook for the Innocent, the Eager, and the Doomed*, both written by Karen Elizabeth Gordon and published by Ticknor & Fields). Everyone participates in the meetings, and we encourage staff to chair portions of the meetings and lead the discussions from time to time.

We believe that staff are our greatest resource and that they need to be trained, developed, and recognized for their skills and contributions. Empowerment is based on a belief in the potential of people. If given the opportunity and encouragement, people can look within and amongst themselves for input, answers, and directions. Empowerment implies that people will be given more input into matters that affect them. Empowered people believe that they can make a difference.

The key to the empowered transcriptionist is a management philosophy of respect, which means listening to, trusting, and supporting each other in our work. This produces a positive work environment where all people work together to achieve common goals. We encourage the people doing the work to make some of the decisions. Who better knows what and how things should be done? We believe that the transcriptionists, working in honest cooperation with each other, can usually make the best decisions about the tasks at hand.

There are definite benefits in this type of work environment. Quality and productivity are very high. Our transcriptionists produce 1500–2000 lines per day and have fun doing it. There is no incentive pay in this hospital, nor do we feel it necessary or even wise. Other positions in the department are not paid according to how many charts they process or code. The incentive for staff is doing the best job they can as members of a team and knowing that they do it very well. We find that sick time and absenteeism are minimal, and we have many long-service employees (10 years and more).

We are proud of our staff and of the quality of work they do.

Reprinted from "Incidental Findings," JAAMT, Vol. 11, No. 2, March-April 1992, pp. 46–47. Copyright 1992, AAMT, Modesto, CA.

Appendix BB

"Value Added" Defined

Pat Forbis, CMT

A t the end of most AAMT educational presentations, speakers encourage the audience to ask questions or share comments. Such was the case at a leadership conference where I was asked to address a variety of issues confronting AAMT's leaders. During the question-and-answer period, a medical transcription service owner asked what is meant by the phrase *value added*. The phrase has appeared frequently in AAMT publications, and I had included it in my presentation, but the individual was uncertain about its definition.

As it is with all question-and-answer periods, limited time did not permit a lengthy response. "The spaces in a transcript," was the reply I gave and, although the answer was appropriate and accurate, it was incomplete. The phrase *value added* provides important marketing information because it tells the customer that quality is a concern of the provider; it assures that if one looks beyond face-value one will find more than was offered in the original bargain.

Webster defines "value" several ways, including ones pertinent to medical transcription:

- *"a fair return or equivalent in goods, services, or money for something exchanged,"*

- *"a numerical quantity that is assigned or is determined by calculation or measurement,"*

- *"something (as a principle or quality) intrinsically valuable or desirable."*

All these definitions are important when describing what added value exists in medical transcription and in AAMT. In fact, there are so many options that it would not be possible to include them in one column.

We could say that the first definition talks about the patient's expectation that s/he will receive accurate, complete, and legible documentation as a part of the services rendered by the physician. It would be fair to say that if the physician is conscientious in terms of patient record documentation, s/he will dictate the report carefully (*value added*) into state-of-the-art equipment (*value added*) to a qualified medical language specialist (*value added*) who will appropriately transcribe it by using the latest available technology (*value added*) and up-to-date resources (*value added*).

The medical transcriptionist then has the opportunity to provide a *value-added* document. A medical language specialist cares enough to place the quality of transcription over the total quantity produced (*value added*). That is not to say that quantity produced is not important; it is to say that each patient's record is grammatically appropriate (*value added*), that spelling is correct (*value added*), that abbreviations have been accurately translated (*value added*), that demographic information is complete (*value added*), and that necessary blanks or potential risks have been flagged for review (*value added*). Oh, yes, spaces DO add value to transcribed reports, especially for those who need to read them. In addition to being spell-checked (*value added*), each document is proofread by a medical language specialist (*value added*).

The physician then reviews the report for content accuracy, clarity, and completeness (*value added*) and signs it as authenticated (*value added*).

By now you may be thinking that what I have described is simply an expectation of how things **should** be done, but there is no doubt that the expertise offered by the qualified medical transcriptionist is a significant value added to patient documentation ... the kind of value that contributes to quality patient care. To prove this point, just watch and listen as healthcare providers attempt to accurately and completely interpret a handwritten patient record.

The second definition speaks to a numerical quantity that is assigned or determined by calculation or measurement. A paradigm shift (*value added*) may be in order before value is added to the current practice of electronically monitoring the work of medical transcriptionists. If data gathering is carefully analyzed by qualified personnel (*value added*), such calculations could be used for market projections that would supply information, products, and services to educators, vendors, service owners, healthcare facilities, and others in our industry.

Medical transcriptionists should individually analyze the measurement of their work at regular intervals (*value added*). By identifying what influences one's production, emphasis on specific continuing education (*value added*) can be placed where needed; i.e., specialty terminology, practicing dictation by physicians who speak English as a second language, skill building. Macros can be designed for standard words or phrases (*value added*).

Studying total quality management (TQM) and continuous quality improvement (CQI) and putting the 14 tenets of quality management into action certainly add value to the work environment. Providing safety in the workplace with ergonomically designed chairs *(value added)*, desks that facilitate ease of keyboard and monitor access *(value added)*, and lighting that protects workers' vision *(value added)* enhances medical transcription recruitment and retention. In addition to improving employee safety, these measures contribute to productivity.

My favorite definition is the last one ... something of intrinsic value. Intrinsic value is that special quality that cannot be easily described. Words are inadequate and pictures fall short of explaining just what it is that makes the value so important. I think medical transcription and you, the medical language specialists who care about quality patient care, add value by

• protecting the patient's right to privacy,

- demonstrating the commitment to production of quality patient documentation,

- seeking continuing education in order to be informed and current on medical narrative style and medical science,

- investigating new products and equipment in order to remain on the cutting edge of technology,

- caring about the healthcare provider by identifying content errors that present potential risks, and doing all this while striving to

  - improve the image of the medical language specialist,
  - upgrade the job classification where necessary,
  - create an independent work environment where necessary,
  - educate others about what medical transcription is and is not,
  - assist educators in preparing worthwhile programs, and
  - mentor newcomers and share your knowledge with your peers.

Many of you do all this and keep an eye to the future by contributing your expertise externally ... authoring, consulting, reviewing, lecturing. Your contributions are your intrinsic value, the *value added* that lends integrity to our profession and all medical transcriptionists. *Value added* ... our list could go on but space is limited.

Medical transcription service owners, physicians and other healthcare providers, supervisors, and others in positions of so-called authority who speak to mere outcome (the finished product) would be well served to consider just what it is that goes beyond bottom line analysis and provides *value added* in our industry. *Value added* in patient documentation is the medical transcriptionist, the medical language specialist.

Reprinted from "Impressions," JAAMT, Vol. 12, No. 5, September-October 1993, pp. 14–15. Copyright 1993, AAMT, Modesto, CA.

Appendix CC

State Names and Abbreviations, Major Cities, and State/City Resident Designations

Note: An asterisk after a city name means it can stand alone in text., i.e., it is not necessary to add the state name following it.

state	abbreviations (stnd)	(USPS)	residents (state or city)	major cities
Alabama	Ala.	AL	Alabamians	
				Birmingham
				Mobile
				Montgomery
Alaska		AK	Alaskans	
				Anchorage*
				Fairbanks
				Juneau
Arizona	Ariz.	AZ	Arizonans	
			Arizonians	
				Phoenix*
				Tucson
Arkansas	Ark.	AR	Arkansans	
			Arkansians	
				Fort Smith
				Little Rock*
California	Calif.	CA	Californians	
				Hollywood*
			Angeleans	Los Angeles*
			Sacramentans	Sacramento
			San Diegans	San Diego*
			San Franciscans	San Francisco*
Colorado	Colo.	CO	Coloradans	
			Coloradoans	
				Colorado Springs
			Denverites	Denver*

state	*abbreviations* (stnd) (USPS)		*residents* (state or city)	*major cities*
Connecticut	Conn.	CT		Bridgeport Hartford New Haven
Delaware	Del.	DE	Delawareans	 Dover
Florida	Fla.	FL	Floridians Floridans Miamians	 Jacksonville Miami* Orlando* Tampa St. Petersburg
Georgia	Ga.	GA	Georgians Atlantans	 Atlanta* Augusta
Hawaii		HI	Hawaiians	Honolulu*
Idaho	Ida.	ID	Idahoans	 Boise
Illinois	Ill.	IL	Illinoisans Illinoians Illinoisians Chicagoans	 Chicago* Springfield
Indiana	Ind.	IN	Indianans Indianians	 Ft. Wayne Indianapolis* South Bend
Iowa	Ia.	IA	Iowans	 Des Moines Sioux City

state	abbreviations		residents	major cities
	(stnd)	(USPS)	(state or city)	
Kansas	Kan.	KS	Kansans	
			Kansas Citians	Kansas City
				Topeka
				Wichita
Kentucky	Ken.	KY	Kentuckians	
				Knoxville
				Lexington
Louisiana	La.	LA	Louisianans	
			Louisianians	
				Baton Rouge
				New Orleans*
				Shreveport
Maine	Me.	ME	Mainers	
				Augusta
				Bangor
				Portland
Maryland	Md.	MD	Marylanders	
				Annapolis
			Baltimoreans	Baltimore*
Massachusetts	Mass.	MA	Bostonians	Boston*
				Springfield
				Worcester
Michigan	Mich.	MI	Michiganders	
			Michiganites	
				Detroit*
				Flint
				Grand Rapids
				Kalamazoo
				Lansing
Minnesota	Minn.	MN	Minnesotans	
				Minneapolis*
				Rochester
				St. Paul

state	abbreviations (stnd) (USPS)		residents (state or city)	major cities
Mississippi	Miss.	MS	Mississipians	Biloxi Gulfport Jackson
Missouri	Mo.	MO	Missourians Kansas Citians	Kansas City* Springfield St. Louis*
Montana	Mont.	MT	Montanans	Billings Butte Great Falls Helena
Nebraska	Neb.	NE	Nebraskans	Grand Island Lincoln Omaha*
Nevada	Nev.	NV	Nevadans Nevadians Las Vegans	Las Vegas* Reno*
New Hampshire	N.H.	NH	New Hampshirites	Concord Manchester
New Jersey	N.J.	NJ	New Jerseyites New Jerseyans	Atlantic City* Camden Newark
New Mexico	N.M.	NM	New Mexicans	Albuquerque* Santa Fe*

state	abbreviations		residents	major cities
	(stnd)	(USPS)	(state or city)	
New York	N.Y.	NY	New Yorkers	
				Albany
				Buffalo
			New Yorkers	New York City*
				Syracuse
North Carolina	N.C.	NC	North Carolinians	
				Charlotte
				Raleigh
				Winston-Salem
North Dakota	N.D.	ND	North Dakotans	
				Bismarck
				Fargo
				Minot
Ohio	O.	OH	Ohioans	
				Cincinnati*
				Cleveland*
				Columbus
Oklahoma	Okla.	OK	Oklahomans	
				Oklahoma City*
				Tulsa*
Oregon	Ore.	OR	Oregonians	
			Portlanders	Portland
Pennsylvania	Penn.	PA	Pennsylvanians	
			Philadelphians	Philadelphia*
				Pittsburgh*
Rhode Island	R.I.	RI	Rhode Islanders	
				Providence
South Carolina	S.C.	SC	South Carolinians	
			Charlestonians	Charleston*
				Columbia
				Greenville

state	*abbreviations* (stnd) (USPS)	*residents* (state or city)	*major cities*
South Dakota	S.D. SD	South Dakotans	
			Rapid City
			Sioux Falls
Tennessee	Tenn. TN	Tennesseans	
			Knoxville
			Memphis*
			Nashville*
Texas	Tex. TX	Texans	
			Austin*
		Dallasites	Dallas*
			El Paso*
		Houstonians	Houston*
		San Antonians	San Antonio*
Utah	UT	Utahans	
		Utahns	
			Salt Lake City*
Vermont	Vt. VT	Vermonters	
			Burlington
Virginia	Va. VA	Virginians	
			Newport News
			Norfolk
			Richmond
			Roanoke
Washington	Wash. WA	Washingtonians	
			Seattle*
			Spokane
			Tacoma
West Virginia	W.Va. WV	West Virginians	
			Charleston
			Huntington
			Wheeling

state	abbreviations		residents	major cities
	(stnd)	(USPS)	(state or city)	
Wisconsin	Wis.	WI	Wisconsonites	
				Green Bay
				Madison
				Milwaukee*
Wyoming	Wy.	WY	Wyomians	
				Casper
				Cheyenne
District of Columbia	D.C.	DC	Washingtonians	Washington

About the Author

Claudia Tessier has been executive director of the American Association for Medical Transcription since 1984. She holds professional credentials as a certified association executive (CAE), certified medical transcriptionist (CMT), and registered record administrator (RRA) and has professional experience in each of these areas as well as in university-level teaching.

Tessier has a BA from San Francisco State University and an MEd from the University of Houston, both in allied health education. In 1993 she was awarded AAMT's first Tessier Award of Excellence and in 1994 was selected Association Executive of the Year by the Northern California Society of Association Executives.

Tessier is a nationally recognized speaker in the fields of association management and medical transcription, where her special interests are quality, the medical and English languages, and the styles and practices of medical transcription. She is the author of *The Surgical Word Book* (W.B. Saunders, 1991), was the primary author of the *Style Guide for Medical Transcription* (AAMT, 1985), serves as editor in chief of the *Journal of AAMT,* has participated in the development of AAMT's Exploring Transcription Practices™ series of modules and videos, and has facilitated numerous AAMT workshops on medical transcription styles and practices.

About AAMT

AAMT is the American Association for Medical Transcription, a national professional association for medical transcriptionists. AAMT's mission is the advancement of medical transcription and the education and development of medical transcriptionists as medical language specialists.

Membership categories include active (medical transcriptionists), as well as associate, student, institutional, and corporate. Membership benefits include the award-winning bimonthly *Journal of the American Association for Medical Transcription* (*JAAMT*); discounts on AAMT meetings and conferences, educational products and logo items, and other services; toll-free access to AAMT's professional staff; and networking opportunities both nationally and through nearly 200 local chapters and state/regional associations throughout the United States and Canada.

AAMT also administers a professional certification program, the *Medical Transcriptionist Certification Program* (MTCP) at AAMT, which awards the CMT (certified medical transcriptionist) professional designation.

For more information on the association and its programs, products, and services, contact

AAMT
PO Box 576187
Modesto, CA 95357-6187

Telephone: 800-982-2182 or 209-551-0883
Fax: 209-551-9317

ORDER FORM

THE AAMT
BOOK OF STYLE FOR
MEDICAL TRANSCRIPTION

PRICES
$49 (AAMT member discounted price*)
$79 (nonmember price)

Please send me ___ copies of *The AAMT Book of Style for Medical Transcription*. My check or money order (U.S. dollars only) is enclosed, or you may bill my credit card.

❑ MasterCard   ❑ VISA   ❑ American Express

Card no._____ Exp. date_____

Cardholder name_____

Authorized signature_____

SHIP TO:

Name_____ AAMT no._____

Address_____

City, state, zip code_____

Day phone (_____)_____ Fax (_____)_____

Prices include standard shipping and handling in the United States and Canada; extra charge for special shipping/handling and/or shipments to other destinations. No refunds. Defective materials replaced if returned to AAMT within 15 days of receipt.

ORDER FROM:
AAMT, P.O. Box 576187, Modesto, CA 95357-6187

CREDIT CARD ORDERS ONLY:
800-982-2182, 209-551-0883, or fax 209-551-9317

*For membership information, contact AAMT at
800-982-2182, 209-551-0883, or fax 209-551-9317